£1.00

A Patient Pharmacist

C000156109

John Atkinson

First Published in 2023 by Blossom Spring Publishing
A Patient Pharmacist © 2023 John Atkinson
ISBN 978-1-7392955-9-2
E: admin@blossomspringpublishing.com
W: www.blossomspringpublishing.com
All rights reserved under International Copyright Law.
Contents and/or cover may not be reproduced without
prior permission of the copyright holder.

Chapters

Foreword

Why?

A good question which can be irrational, irritating, inquisitive, intriguing, imposing and sometimes impossible to answer.

Why the Title "A Patient Pharmacist"?

Simply because I have been both a patient (having undergone 50+ general anaesthetic procedures/operations) and a fully qualified Pharmacist (registered 1980 to 2008).

Why Write a Book?

People say that men don't talk, but they can write.

To share some life experiences and trauma. A tribute to Carol, wife and absolute "rock" of 41 years and to all the healthcare professionals (involved in my treatment) expertise and dedication.

If this book can inspire just one person to seek help for medical or mental timely intervention, then it has been a success (in my eyes).

In this book I will try and cover, with pragmatism, humility and sometimes gallows humour, all that has befallen my wife Carol and me, as well as some career anecdotes as a pharmacist together with my Middlesbrough background history and some early memories.

Why Us?

- Shared loss of a child
- life threatening medical diagnoses and treatment
- redundancy and early retirement

Just a tale of ordinary, normal people living an ordinary, normal and sometimes unlucky life (and yet I'll let you be the judge of that).

Chapter 1

Boro Boys
(Early Memories)

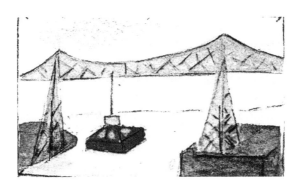

According to the poem "Monday's Child" (published in 1838 by an unknown writer), *"Fridays' child is loving and giving"*.

On Friday 11th April 1958 I was born at "Ardencaple", Lothian Road, Middlesbrough which was a private maternity nursing home (established 1912 and closed in 1964, due to lack of support leaving no private maternity beds in Middlesbrough) the second child of my parents Barrie and Beatrice (Betty), who lived in Ruby Street (also in Middlesbrough). My dad told me that I was born there so that I was in Yorkshire and would therefore qualify to play cricket for Yorkshire (who at that period in time only took on players born within the county). Or maybe, it was because my brother (Stephen) was born (two and a half years earlier) in my grandad and nanna Chester's front room in Pine Street, Cargo Fleet,

Middlesbrough and they did not want to experience that situation again. Both, my dad and his dad (Grandad) were also born in Middlesbrough but my mam was born (1934) in Sandown on the Isle of Wight (nee Chester).

How was it that my mam, her sister Sheenagh and my nanna (Rosina Chester, born 1913), who were all born on the Isle of Wight ended up in Middlesbrough?

My grandad (Albert Chester, born Middlesbrough 1913), at the tender age of 14 and a half pretended that he was 16 and joined the army, initially as a bugler in the Royal Horse Artillery Gun Troop, and then also as a Queen's Trumpeter.

He was stationed around several ports in the South of England and was the Chief Gunnery Officer in charge of the anti-aircraft battery situated on the Needles on the Isle of Wight.

He gained the rank of Lieutenant and fought in World War Two campaigns and was the Adjutant (a military officer who acts as an administrative assistant to a senior officer) of a troop ship which was sent to Tripoli, Libya as part of the Western Desert Force.

He was in charge of the gun battery at the Siege of Tobruk, pounding the German and Italian Axis forces of Rommel. During this combat campaign he received a battlefield promotion to Captain. Returning from this campaign his ship was sunk by a German U boat around the heel of Italy and yet he managed to survive and be rescued.

After World War Two he was demobbed and, as there was no employment in the South, he gained a job as a caretaker at Hugh Bell School in Middlesbrough and so moved back to Cargo Fleet with my mam, nanna and aunty, and of course some time later my mam met my dad.

I have only a limited memory of Ruby Street, as we

left when I was around three to four years of age. I can, however, remember that it was an old Victorian two up two down terraced house and I shared a bedroom with my brother. He had a double bed and I was in a cot next to it and I vividly recall the bottom dropping out of the cot constantly and waking me on many occasions. Bath times, usually once a week on a Sunday, were taken in a tin bath in front of the coal fire in the kitchen/diner and I was, always, the last in the bath after my dad and my brother (Stephen) and the water was inevitably tepid and perhaps not the cleanest.

My grandad (Joseph Atkinson) was born (1894) in Middlesbrough and lived at Kildare Street, and at the age of 14 he left school and became a horse drawn delivery wagon driver for the Co-Operative.

1914 saw the outbreak of World War One and he volunteered to fight and joined the East Yorkshire Regiment (a line infantry regiment of the British Army). He fought in, and survived, the trenches of the Battle of the Somme (at Morval) between July and November 1916. More than three million men fought in this battle, with one million killed or wounded (one of the deadliest battles in human history).

In 1917 he fought in Belgium at the Battle of Passchendaele (The Third Battle of Ypres, at which there were up to 400,000 British casualties) and it was here that shrapnel shattered his leg and left him invalided. He was stretchered to the Casualty Clearing Station (Field Hospital) at Ypres, and his wound was probably treated with Dakin's antibacterial solution or Dakin-Carel solution and others such as sodium hypochlorite, boric acid and tincture of iodine with daily dressing changes.

The most frequent causes of death in World War One were not mainly related to gunshot wounds but rather to fractures, tetanus and septic complications of infectious diseases in this pre-antibiotic era and it is due to this nursing care that he survived.

He was then transferred to a hospital in Dorset, England and spent 12 months there for further treatment and recuperation.

Every year until he died (in 1971) he sent a Christmas card to the nurse in Dorset who nursed him through his injuries. He managed to work as a wages clerk at Cochrane Iron Foundry of North Ormesby, Middlesbrough who produced cast-iron pipes, railway chairs and large iron castings for worldwide distribution and to facilitate this had their own wharf on the bank of the Tees (in sight of the Tees Transporter Bridge). Ill health exacerbated by a perforated duodenal ulcer enforced early retirement at the age of just 49.

My grandad Joseph always seemed old and frail to me and was a very quiet man who never spoke about his experiences (like many veterans who experienced such horrors), though he did let me play with his tin soldiers, World War One medals and military Dinky toys without much comment, for which I had fond memories.

My dad (born 1933) had two older brothers, Uncle Bill (Joseph William, born 1920) and Geoffrey (born 1928). Unfortunately I never knew Geoffrey as he died in 1943 as a result of kidney trouble.

Uncle Bill is now 102 years old, living in Jesmond, Newcastle upon Tyne and I think, as a Boro Boy born and bred, that part of his story should also be shared here.

In 1940 he volunteered for RAF Aircrew duties and during World War Two he flew, and survived, 20 day/night missions over France and Germany as a Lancaster Bomber navigator for No. 61 squadron.

Flight Lieutenant J W Atkinson DFC, was awarded the Distinguished Flying Cross in 1945 and his service story can be found on the website www.no-50-and-no-61-

squadrons-association.co.uk/veterans-album/f-lt-j-w-atkinson-dfc/.

I quote his own words on receipt of this medal: *"I was surprised to receive some telegrams congratulating me on being awarded the DFC for my tour with 61 squadron. Apparently, it had appeared in the London Gazette sometime in August 1945. And it had reached the local paper in Middlesbrough. There was a small reference in one of the editions. I received the actual medal through the post some months later in the summer of 1946, with a printed communication from George VI."*

These stories deserve to be retold *"Lest we forget"* and I am proud of the service and sacrifice given by my Boro Boy relatives during both World Wars.

Back to my dad (Barrie), who after completing his post war national service in the RAF became a steelworks clerk at Redpath Dorman Long Limited in Redcar, Middlesbrough.

Dorman Long (by1914) employed 20,000 people and, together with the Cleveland Bridge Company, were responsible for the construction and manufacture for the harbour bridges in Sydney and Auckland, river crossings across Africa and projects such as London's Lambeth Bridge, the Tyne Bridge connecting Newcastle and Gateshead and also Middlesbrough's Newport Bridge.

In 1961 Dorman Long opened a factory on the Aycliffe Industrial Estate, Newton Aycliffe, and my dad became its Sales/Production Manager, later to become General Manager.

The factory was equipped with two coating lines and built-in curing ovens for the production of double-sided PVC painted steel sheets. These sheets were then shaped producing profile sheets up to 36ft long for the construction industry.

As a result we moved from Middlesbrough to Newton

Aycliffe.

This was not to be the end of my time in Middlesbrough as nearly every weekend we visited both sets of grandparents, but more about that shortly, after a little background on Newton Aycliffe.

In 1941 a Royal Ordnance factory (ROF Aycliffe) operated 24 hours a day producing shells for World War Two and by 1945 had produced over 700 million bullets and countless other munitions, with the workers (some 6000) being mainly women and known as the "Aycliffe Angels".

These workers and their families needed somewhere to live and so the Aycliffe Development Corporation proposed a new town, and called it, surprisingly, Newton Aycliffe.

Lord Beveridge adopted this new town as the flagship of his new welfare state in which he envisaged a "classless" town, where manager and mechanic would live next door to each other in council houses.

In his words, Newton Aycliffe was to be a "paradise for housewives" with houses grouped around greens, so children could play safely away from the roads.

It was within this context that we moved into our "Bousefield Crescent" council house (all houses were council with no private developments until the Margaret Thatcher era). As a child it was so exciting as in 1961 new houses were rapidly being built to replace the earlier pre-fabricated houses.

In fact the builders hut was opposite our house and I could often be found chattering with the builders and joining them for a cuppa tea served from their white enamel tea urns.

Some newspapers in the '60s were very critical of the town even calling it *"The Town That Has No Heart"* and *"perfect planning and perfect monotony ... nothing to do and nowhere to go"*, even criticising the town centre, *"12 small shops. A few more half-built and a keen, cold wind".* One youth reported in 1964, *"It's a dump really. There is nothing to do."*

However, this was offset by the Northern Despatch paper which reported *"an endless stream of clubs, trips and shows organised by the people of Newton Aycliffe".* It was exciting to me though, due to having plenty of friends and space to play together.

I attended Vane Road Infants and Junior school and would walk, daily, from our house (in my grey shorts, maroon jumper and school cap) with my brother and friends. In fact short trousers were the "order of the day" until big school at the ripe old age of 11 years.

I only got into a few mishaps at school, as in that I only received the "cane" form of corporal punishment twice, once for throwing snowballs! And, secondly, for squirting other kids with water from a water pistol. Well in truth not exactly a water pistol but rather in the form of 50ml or 100ml unused, clean plastic syringes (which could deliver with some force) acquired by a friend!

1969 was a memorable last year in school for several reasons, firstly I was in the final year school choir and can still remember, today, the words sung to such songs as "Men of Harlech", "The Song of the Western Men" (Trelawny's song), "The Skye Boat Song", "Busy Doing Nothing" (Bing Crosby) and "Little Arrows" (Leapy Lee).

Secondly, we all sat transfixed in the assembly hall watching hazy black and white pictures of the moon landing on the school's TV, it was 21st July 1969. Then, after school, I continued to watch it with the rest of our family on the rented "Rediffusion" TV.

Lastly, I had been selected, upon assessment by the teaching staff (the old 11+ examinations had just been disbanded), to attend Ferryhill Technical Grammar School.

In the 1970s Newton Aycliffe underwent a rapid growth, together with a Recreation Centre (complete with sports hall, swimming pool and squash courts), Municipal Golf Course, Angling pool and a Boy's Club on Burnhill Way. In 1978 Boots The Chemists opened a large store (which in later years myself and my nephew became employed with). Then in 1979 a Fine Fare supermarket opened together with a weekly open-air market and the Aycliffe Development Corporation also began selling its council houses and a project to convert houses with flat roofs (and put an end to Aycliffe's "little boxes") began. All this development was missed by me as, in 1971, we moved to Darlington.

My brother and dad still live in Newton Aycliffe (after returning there) and my brother's two children attended Vane Road school and now my nephew's children (third generation) are also attending there.

My mam currently also lives in a Newton Aycliffe nursing home (secure Dementia Unit), where she has been resident for at least four years now suffering from Vascular Dementia (a cruel condition). For the last three years she has not recognised me and the rest of the family and we try and visit whenever we can (although Covid has prevented this on many an occasion). My dad used to visit her every day and is now only able to manage three or four days a week, it is so heart wrenching for all.

Back to my childhood visits to both sets of grandparents in "Ironopolis" (a name Middlesbrough came to be known as, due to 40 or so blast furnaces and the extraction of iron ore from the nearby Eston Hills). These visits mainly happened on Saturdays when Middlesbrough FC played at home.

Visits also included seeing aunts and uncles, of which

there were dozens as it seemed that every relative of my parents' age and above, who wasn't a grandparent, was called Aunt or Uncle. My parents aunts and uncles (my great aunts and great uncles), and my parents cousins, all simply became known as Uncle or Aunty and so clouds my recollections of who is actually who. I'm sure this is the same for most families of that era and even to this day.

Saturday trips to Grandad A's (Kildare Street) followed a regular routine of a fish and chip lunch, then a couple of beers (at the "Westminster Hotel" pub on Parliament Road) for my dad and grandad before they walked just along a couple of streets to Ayresome Park, to watch our beloved Middlesbrough football club play. Up to the age of six, I was deemed too young to go and so instead went with my mam and grandma along Linthorpe Road into Middlesbrough town centre. Shops visited included the Co-Op, in order to accumulate as well as spend the "Divvy" (dividend loyalty bonus), the Penny Bazaar (otherwise known as Marks and Spencers) and an obligatory stop at Rea's Ice Cream Parlour for a toasted marshmallow together with a "lemon-top" ice cream or an ice cream floater.

The Rea ice cream empire, at its peak in the 1970s, employed more than 200 people and had 21 snack bars across Teeside. Rock star Chris, son of owner Casmillo, publicised his debut single "So Much Love" by being pictured with a Stop Me And Buy One bike. Chris Rea lived above the ice cream parlour beside Albert Park and could be regularly heard practising on his guitar. His famous hits of course include "On the beach", The Road to Hell", "Auberge", "Driving Home for Christmas", "Let's Dance", etc. and he has produced 25 solo albums, a true Boro Boy rock legend.

Then it was back to Kildare Street so that my grandma

could watch the horse racing and *World of Sport Wrestling* (watching such names as Jackie Palo and Giant Haystacks perform). Tea was nearly always a ham or salmon and cucumber sandwich followed by a fresh cream brandy snap and or Chocolate Ginger Thins (both from St Michael i.e. M&S), which were Grandma and Grandad's favourites. After the age of six, I also went to the football matches along with my brother and stood in the "Boy's end", dressed in our hand knitted red and white scarves and pom pom hats making a noise with our wooden football rattles and shouting "Boro Boys Boro Boys we are here whoa ho, whoa ho".

The Kildare Street house was on a cobbled road of Victorian terraced houses and boasted a back yard and outside "Privy". I always thought that going to the loo was a spooky adventure especially in the cold dark depths of winter when the only heating and light was provided by a tea-light, paraffin burner (Boom Boom Esso Blue) and your torch. Loo paper consisted of either strips of newspaper or if you were lucky then slippy "Izal" toilet paper (rolls or boxes). You tended not to ponder too long there. What would today's kids make of it all, I wonder?

Mondays were always washing days for Grandma and washing was done using a wash board, tub and poss stick (wooden dolly) and a hand wringer, which were later replaced by a twin washer/spinner and electric wringer. This remained to be the order of our Middlesbrough visits until my grandma died (suddenly at the washing up sink) in 1969 and my Grandad A (until his death in 1971) went to live with my Uncle Bill, in Newcastle upon Tyne.

Grandad C and Nanna's house in Pine Street, Cargo Fleet, Middlesbrough was again a Victorian terraced house on a cobbled road (which was a cul-de-sac with a half brick wall at the end topped with corrugated iron sheet). From the street and back yard you could see the glow and smell the sulphur of the constantly lit blast furnaces of Cargo Fleet.

Because it was a "Dead-end" street we regularly kicked a ball around and played games such as Hopscotch, "Wallee" and "Kerby". In Kerby, two kids stood on opposite kerbs of the road/street facing each other and the aim of the game was to throw the ball across the street to try and hit the opposite side of the pavement kerb. If you missed the kerb, the other kid took their turn. If the ball bounced back to the thrower you were awarded a point. If a player managed to catch the ball during the bounce back they would be awarded additional points. a range of points was also awarded for different throws such as a blind throw over your head as it was much harder to execute.

With "Wallee" we used to chalk a target on the "dead-end wall" and score points, very much like an archery target except by kicking a ball (any football or tennis ball) at the target from different distances and angles. We also drew goalposts on the wall and had a proper game of football. We played other games (also enjoyed in the playground) such as "Tig", in which one kid chased another and tried to touch them. Whoever was touched then became "it" and they became the chaser.

Another similar "Tig" game was British Bulldog in which one player attempted to intercept other players who must run from one designated area to another, and often with large numbers of kids as neighbouring streets joined in. It was all so safe, due to the street being a cul-de-sac and cars were rare or even non-existent.

At the opposite end of the street was the trolleybus terminus and we used to watch with fascination the sparks that were emitted from the overhead lines and the bus gantry connection; an operative with a long pole could often be seen disconnecting this connection so that the bus could change lines and/or direction.

The Middlesbrough trolleybus system opened in 1919 (and was unusual in the UK, in that it was a completely new rail-less system that didn't replace any existing tramway network and did not close until 1971). The three routes served by this system included North Ormesby, Cargo Fleet, South Bank, Normanby, Grangetown and Eston.

As a family we travelled many times on these dark or pale/mid-green with a cream roof, as near to Middlesbrough town centre as we could, although that involved either a good walk or catching a standard "United" bus from the Smeaton Street terminus. It was fun to climb the stairs to the top deck where a conductor would issue a ticket by cranking a handle on the silver machine hanging around his neck.

Me and my brother both wanted to climb the Middlesbrough Transporter Bridge and venture along its walkway high above the River Tees; however, my dad was afraid of heights and so Uncle Wilf stepped in.

The Middlesbrough Transporter Bridge, with its light blue livery and appearance, is such an icon for the area. It was built between 1910 and 1911 at a cost of £68,026 6s 8d (around £8 million at today's value) to replace the "Hugh Bell" and "Erimus" steam ferry services. The transporter was chosen so that a road system of crossing the river could stop the ferry's effect on the river navigation. When working it carried a travelling "car" or "gondola", suspended below the fixed structure, across the river in 90 seconds. The gondola could carry 200 people, nine cars, or six cars and one minibus. The bridge connects Middlesbrough, on the South bank, to Stockton on Tees, on the north bank, and carries the A178 road from Middlesbrough to Hartlepool.

As a structure its longest span is 851 ft (259m) and the

clearance below is 160ft (49m) and what a view (from the upper walkway at such a height) of Middlesbrough and the Tees it was.

Grandad C subsequently changed jobs, still as a caretaker but instead at a special educational needs school in Redcar, and it came with an on-site tied cottage and, consequently, Redcar then became a focus of our visits.

As we visited Redcar at weekends, no students were on site and so we were able to play in the school playground upon which stood a non-operational Austin A40 car for us to "drive".

My brother Stephen and I used to pretend that we were racing and rallying the car around a racetrack like Jim Clark (a Formula One racing driver who won two world championships and also competed in sports, and touring cars and the Indianapolis 500). This simulated racing was imaginative play and kept us occupied for many an hour and indeed kept us dry when it rained.

However, we longed for "live" racing and so we built our very own two-man racing car in the form of a "bogie" (not something up your nose, but rather a home-made wagon). This was lovingly constructed using a wooden box, planks, four old pram wheels, nuts, bolts, a piece of washing line to steer with and completed with a brake. We could often be seen speeding downhill (just like adrenaline junkies, and Jim Clark) from Grandad's house onto the streets and roads of Redcar.

In June 1964 we holidayed with Grandad C and Nanna at Butlin's Holiday Camp, Filey, on the beautiful rugged North Yorkshire Coast. We arrived, by Grandad's car, which we parked in a large compound, within a fenced-off parking area (much like an airport car park today) near the entrance to the camp. Immediately we were met and greeted by "Redcoats" (the entertainment staff) and it all seemed so magical, not unlike an early version of today's theme parks.

The camp buildings and facilities were all brightly painted in blues, yellows, white and of course red. It was also so exciting to be taken to our chalet, along the main avenue, on "Puffing Billy", a road train, which went everywhere on site.

I use the word chalet reservedly as it was more like a brightly coloured beach hut, with bunk beds and paper thin walls (through which you could hear all the "shenanigans" in the adjacent chalets).

I remember swimming in the outdoor and indoor heated pools with my flippers and rubber goggles (which had the appearance of those worn by welders).

There was a chairlift, helter-skelter, boating lake, fun fair (with numerous types of spinning rides), a "Peter Pan" railway, access to the beach, a Big Wheel, and even a car road track. What more could a child desire? Great fun was had by all.

Entertainment (provided by the Red Coats) was certainly the order of the day with competitions such as "knobbly" knees, beauty pageants, singing and painting. Evening entertainment, provided for the adults, included dancing, cabaret, musical and magician shows and of course the bars, "Gaiety" and "Sportsman's"

The PA and Tannoy System was regularly making announcements, playing music and calling guests to lunch and breakfast with words like "Good morning, campers, breakfast is now being served in the canteen". Canteen it certainly was, in that it resembled a massive military mess hall and so noisy and loud.

Anyone who has watched the TV series *Hi-de-Hi* will certainly have been shown a glimpse of life at Butlin's.

Butlin's Filey was a 10,000-capacity camp – a former wartime military training base called RAF Hunmanby Moor – opened in 1945 and closed in 1983 (primarily due to the advent of cheap holidays abroad). It was served by its own railway branch and station (Filey Holiday Camp railway station) which closed in 1977 due to greater car ownership. Part of the camp has subsequently been replaced by "Primrose Valley" holiday park and the adjacent "The Bay Filey" holiday resort.

On return from this holiday I remember being driven past Middlesbrough Maternity Hospital (referred to as "Parkside" due to its location by the side of the town's Albert Park) and seeing my mam and dad in the bay window holding up my baby brother, David. Unfortunately that was the first and last time that I saw him as he died shortly afterwards. I do not know the tragic circumstances as it was never discussed, perhaps because I was so young or that in later life it brought too many tragic memories in that grief was dealt with differently then.

Whilst we lived in Newton Aycliffe, during school holidays we often stayed with aunts and uncles and grandparents, in order that my mam and dad were able to continue working.

Unfortunately my grandad Chester died at Christmas 1968, due to illness following an earlier stroke yet he just managed to meet his new baby granddaughter, my sister Jane. My nanna then went to live in Mirfield, West Yorkshire with Uncle Graham (my mam's brother) who had moved there upon leaving the army to become a mechanic on some of the world's largest mobile digger machines, trucks and cranes.

Uncle Graham served in the army (REME) and following tours in the jungles of Borneo became based at Ripon North Yorkshire, where again my brother and I visited for holidays.

I can remember "tripping around" with Uncle Graham, as a pillion passenger on his Norton Commando motorbike, trying to lean over at the correct moments as we tore around tight bends in the road (more adrenaline rush).

Other school holidays were spent in Branston, near Lincoln, at my uncle Richard's ("Dick" Chester) house, which also served as a stopover point for family holidays to the Isle of Wight.

Branston was close to RAF Waddington and most days we saw, and heard, Vulcan Bombers flying overhead. By 1961, three squadrons of Vulcans (Black Bucks) were stationed at Waddington and remained there until 1984 and, due to modifications for air-to air refuelling, undertook the bomber attack of Argentine positions at Port Stanley airport during the Falklands war. Today Waddington is one of the RAF's busiest operational airfields, supporting operations all around the world including Remotely Piloted Air Systems using the Reaper (MQ-9A), used in Afghanistan.

It was also at Branston that we regularly watched Richard playing cricket, learnt many playing card games (such as *Stop the Bus*, *Whist*, *Rummy*, *Contract Whist* and *Chase The Ace*) a very popular pastime with many of my Lincoln relatives. We visited the Lincolnshire seaside resort of Mablethorpe, which had a small fairground and traditional amusement arcades but not in the same league as Butlin's Filey, Blackpool or Scarborough. It did, though, have a very long sandy beach with sand dunes, down which you could roll and roll and roll.

Richards's mam (Aunty Edith) also lived in the village in a large house and garden overlooking fields (a sharp contrast to Cargo Fleet). Playing in her garden was an adventure, both feeding the chickens and generally exploring like a regular little David Bellamy, just enjoying nature. The garden also had a disused air raid shelter and an old outside Victorian compost toilet, it was this latter item that fascinated me as a child. It consisted of what resembled a plank (in which were cut several horseshoe shaped and sculptured holes) sat on a wooden box with a long lid. These earth closets remained common in rural areas well into the Edwardian era and incorporated a hopper which dispensed dry, granular clay, (sometimes also together with sawdust, ashes and earth) on top of the waste, into the box. This desiccated the waste and reduced smells. When the box was full the earth and waste could be removed for disposal elsewhere in the garden, fertilising the roses and vegetables. Fortunately for us townies this was no longer in use and the house had a flush loo.

As I write this, in my brain is an image of the man of the house trying to have solitude sitting and reading the paper when his wife joins him on the adjacent hole in the "Netty", asking him how his work day had gone and telling him of her day's events!

Matches at Lincoln City Football Club, at which Richard was Club Secretary, were also very much enjoyed. Richard was also to become the only club secretary to serve both Sheffield United and Sheffield Wednesday (1984-1986).

It was during these appointments that he asked my dad to scout players at the North East Clubs and provide player match reports. As a consequence along I went, with him (and stood on many a terrace in all weathers), to reserve team matches at Sunderland, Middlesbrough and Newcastle as well as first team games at Hartlepool and Darlington to perhaps find that elusive big signing.

Chapter 2

"Big School"

Back to 1969 when we still lived in Newton Aycliffe and I had to travel, daily, the six miles to Ferryhill Grammar School. This was achieved by catching one of the four available morning school buses run by OK Motor Services (based in Bishop Auckland) all having a distinctive maroon and cream livery.

Which of the first three single decker buses you caught depended on the time you made it to the pick-up point on Central Avenue (the nearest). However, if you were a little bit late (which occurred often, and sometimes on purpose as a challenge) you had to walk further into town and catch the double decker. This literally meant jumping on board at the very last minute, as it was moving off, and catching hold of the bus deck pole, great fun.

Returning home I nearly always caught the first one available unless staying after lessons for some particular reason, and then you had to walk into town and catch a service bus and pay the fare. School homework was mostly and hurriedly completed on the bus (which may also account for my writing being a scrawl then and now).

Ferryhill, as its name suggests, was built on a hill (a magnesian limestone escarpment) and the school was on the road from Ferryhill, which ran along the top of this escarpment to the village of Kirk Merrington. The school was frequently battered by strong winds and its twin parallel blocks pointed into the prevailing wind, acting like a wind tunnel causing the school doors to frequently blow off.

During my time there it seemed to snow a lot, with drifts often being two to three foot deep into which (often only dressed in plimsoles with no socks, shorts and gym shirt) we were dumped (as brass monkeys) for school cross country, or even to play rugby by the giant of a PE teacher, Mr Glasper.

Mr Glasper was also a professional wrestler known as "Ray Diamond" (and The White Angel) and was regularly seen fighting (performing) in Middlesbrough and the North East. No doubt my grandma watched him many times, and for any other wrestling fans his interesting life story can be found on the British Wrestling History website *Heritage* at **www.wrestlingheritage.co.uk/ray-diamond**.

The school bus always seemed to manage to make it through the snow, and it makes you laugh how nowadays (due to health and safety) that schools appear to shut at even the hint of a dusting of snow.

I often missed the school bus home due to practise for the school's drama production or sports activities such as football, cricket and swimming after lessons and consequently had to undertake the long march into town. Not only did I play cricket for my year groups but I also volunteered as a "Scorer" (recording every ball bowled and every run scored in a special scorebook) for the older teams.

Lessons, preceded by a morning school assembly (with all the teachers in their black gowns just like Harry Potter), were all very traditional (including mathematics which was taught using the "proof" system). Once in school, you were not allowed to use bags, rucksacks or satchels and had to carry all text books, work books, pen and pencil cases, even piled up with your sports gear, between lessons, This of course proved a challenge on

21

those wet, windy and snowy days.

Corporal punishment also prevailed here, though I was only on the receiving end of the cane once whilst there. I had just finished my Maths exam early, closed my exam papers, placed my writing implements on top and sat bored. So with plenty of time to spare I pulled out my latest Marvel comic (from the floor) and started to read. The teacher went "ballistic" and there and then gave me three whacks on my open palm in front of the class. Not only did it hurt but it was also so degrading.

Anyway I survived Grammar School and at the end of the second year started at Longfield Comprehensive School following my parents move, firstly, to Glebe Road and then, secondly, North Road, Darlington. It was of course here that I was to meet Carol and we became an item, but just a few tales before then.

Nicknames were of course popular at school and here I became known as Nax (formerly Acky at Ferryhill and then Atto at University) others were called such names as Boz, Jike, Carrots and Nobby (the reason for his nickname cannot be told here).

Pupils at the school were divided into houses, both mine and Carol's was called "Cheshire" after Leonard Cheshire and represented in sports by the colour blue. I represented Cheshire in swimming, cricket (also for school and town) as well as football (goal keeper). These were also enjoyed out of school together with lawn tennis and squash. Even though the school had its own athletics track I had a dislike of running for its own sake and much preferred team sports.

When we moved to North Road our new house was next door to a school friend (also previously at Ferryhill) called Carrots. Today he is known to me as Marty Baby (called as such because he calls me John Boy, after the character in the TV series *The Waltons*). We remain very good friends today and keep in regular contact (he now lives in Birmingham and did so when we were later also, to live in The Midlands).

In our early teens we also, together, experienced the introduction to the world of work in the form of potato picking, tomato picking and even "Snaggering". Potato (Tattie) picking always occurred in the October half-term and involved a tractor with a flat-bed trailer (from Barkers' farm) arriving each morning at Harrowgate Hill to pick up a bunch of us kids waiting in line (we, like the Tatties, were hand-picked depending on how old we looked and our position in the line) to take us to Beaumont Hill. No seat belts or health and safety in those days as we all just sat on the deck of the flat-bed as it drove up the main A1 road.

Sticks and string marked out an area (patch) the length of which was determined by us kids' ability and inevitably lengthened as the day/s progressed. We scooped up the potatoes into a plastic basket when the tractor/digger ploughing along the row had passed by. You had to scoop up all the potatoes before the tractor made its next run. Once the baskets were full the Tatties were poured into old oil drum barrels which were then picked up by another tractor into another trailer.

The back-breaking eight-hour-long days seemed endless with just short morning and afternoon "piece" breaks, and a longer one for lunch. It was a stroke of luck if you were able to sit on square bales of hay, scattered about the field, rather than simply on your basket. Lunch often consisted of a jam or Spam butty together with a packet of crisps and an apple, packed in greaseproof paper by Mam.

The weather in late October could be very inclement to say the least, and could alternate between persistent and heavy rain downpours (driven on a strong autumnal wind and interspersed with sunny spells). The worst weather usually occurred early in the morning in the form of a low, cold and soaking mist. It all seemed worth it though at the end of the day when you received your cash in a little brown paper envelope and then returned back home to the welcome of a warm bath.

Sometimes, once you became well known to the farmer, you moved up into the world and you were allowed to work on the "Vulcan" potato harvester. This was a blessing as it involved standing (not bending) under a canopy cover which kept out the elements. The harvester scooped up the potatoes and you stood on a platform (accommodating up to six people) alongside a conveyor belt and threw out any stones that were mixed with the Tatties.

Having experienced this work, we decided to try or hands at turnip/swede picking otherwise known as "Snaggering". This was a complete contrast, although it was also "piece work", i.e. you got paid for the number of rows of turnips picked (at the rate of just 50p a row). There was no hourly rate for number of hours worked, it was only based on the rows.

You were given a heavy, and very sharp, machete knife and shown a few basic rules (hardly health and safety again). Picking actually involved pulling the snagger from the ground and then chopping off the top and bottom growth with said machete. This I attempted to do by placing the swede on the ground and then swinging the machete to chop off its top and bottom. However, this was slow and unproductive. I remember an old farm hand coming up to us showing us his left hand with three missing fingers and uttering the words, "Tha'll never make much money, laddie, until tha've lost a poke or two." Apparently the quickest method was to pull the swede out of the ground with your left hand and whilst still holding it, with the machete in your right hand, chop off the bottom followed swiftly and decisively by the top.

After a full day's work I had only amassed the grand sum of 75p, my brother managed two whole pounds. Consequently we never returned to work this field.

In the summer of 1970 Marty and I decided to try our hand at tomato picking.

The tomato picking work was undertaken at Merrybent greenhouse nurseries which, at six miles from home, was reached by cycling through the west end of Darlington, passing the Broken Scar waterworks en route. All day harvesting tomatoes from the vines in the greenhouses, at the height of summer, was extremely hot and humid (a far cry indeed, from a cold and wet October). The song that reminds me of this time, played all the time over the greenhouse radio, is "In the Summertime" *by* Mungo Jerry.

I then progressed to my first Saturday job which was on a greengrocery stall within Darlington Indoor market for a princely sum of £1.50 per day. It involved an early start as my role was to collect the fresh fruit and vegetables from the wholesalers situated in the market cellar, and then to dress the stall.

I used to load a sack barrow with up to six sacks of potatoes, swedes, carrots or boxes of cauliflowers, apples, oranges etc. or indeed any combination thereof. The barrow then (with a great amount of force) had to be wheeled up the steep embankment of Tubwell Row to the front entrance of the market. Perhaps building muscles like Ray Diamond.

The cauliflowers were trimmed, potatoes brushed and apples were polished before joining the rest of the fruit and vegetables dressed on the market stall. The owner had a real sense of pride in the presentation so that the stall was attractive to customers and in competition with the numerous other fruit and veg stalls.

Once this was achieved the job was to serve the customers efficiently and politely. Big white weighing (Avery) scales were used from which you could read both the weight and its cost from a manual scale on the needle hand. The cost of each item was then written down on a brown paper bag and the total sum to be charged, calculated using mental arithmetic (no calculators or cash register to do the sums). Payment and change given were then simply into and from a metal cash box.

A hour for lunch was taken, for which I would purchase a "savoury" from Middleton's café stall. This savoury consisted of a soft white bread bun containing a mixture of slowly browned fried onions, sausage meat and pepper which was something of a "Darlingtonian" institution. I would often meet Carol outside British Home Stores (where she also had a Saturday job) during this lunch break.

I then managed to secure a job in the food hall of the prestigious "Binns" store (which was to Darlington as Harrod's was to London) and the job was more varied and initially involved pricing and stacking shelves of upmarket tins of fruit in booze, cakes in tins, teas and coffee tins and even caviar. Progression was to, firstly, move onto the delicatessen counter where I sold everything from pate, cheese, Ayrshire roll bacon and Binns' own home boiled cooked ham bacon.

My job was to bone the raw ham, remove the bones, roll and tie it up with string using a special slip-knot. The hams were then placed in plastic sealed bags put into a large industrial water bath and steamed until cooked, then cooled and then placed in walk-in fridges.

Secondly, I moved onto the bakery counter which meant an earlier start as the various breads, cobs, (including many a different shape, style, size and colour of buns), cooked pies, pasties, sausage rolls and all manner of cakes and fancies had to be brought from the bakery and displayed on counter before the store opened.

The rest of the day involved selling to the customers lined up in a seemingly never-ending queue. Late afternoon was the best time of the day as we had to return dozens and dozens of bakery trays (via large wooden trolleys and many journeys) to the bakery ready for the evening baking shift. The bakery was situated several floors up, at the rear of the store, accessed by a walkway that was remote from the rest of the store and so beyond the eyes of the management or supervisory teams.

The ovens were constantly alight, and so, as we stacked the trays, we would help ourselves to uncooked meat pies from the fridge, place them on a long wooden handled spatula and into the oven to bake. The bakery radio was turned on quietly (so that we could hear anybody approaching via the lift and walkway) whilst we listened to the football results and feasted ourselves on the tasty, hot and freshly baked pies.

One day I was serving on the bakery counter when a couple of local thugs strolled up and shouted at another Saturday lad, serving next to me, "Hey, Goldy, who are you looking at?" (He had a couple of gold caps on his two front teeth) to which he replied, "Nothing when I look at your ugly mugs." Then all hell broke loose and the two thugs jumped over the counter and started to attack him, and bread and cakes were scattered all over to the bewilderment of staff and customers alike.

Fortunately, standing in the queue were two plain clothed policeman, who together with store security staff handcuffed the offenders, took them down to the fridges and held them there until the local police came and arrested them. Apparently the offenders were from a rival area of Darlington as that of the Saturday staff member and there was some history between them involved.

Darlington, like many Northern towns during the 1970s, experienced hooliganism, gangs and street fighting. As young teenagers rival gangs existed within different areas of the town, and even between neighbouring streets with fights occurring. There were rivalries between schools and youth clubs and you had to take care not to overstep a boundary, be savvy at times and be ready to run to avoid an attack.

I leave the final word on this to the words of a local newspaper reporter in the Northern Echo, dated October 17th, 1973, head line: ***"Reign of Terror by Clockwork Orange Gang"***

"Warfare between youths armed with knives, bottles and Clockwork Orange-type walking sticks have been causing a hell of a problem in Darlington, claimed a local youth worker. Mass gang warfare involving 60 or 70 youths being involved and centred around various youth clubs and involving up to five gangs has been reported. Albert Road, Brinkburn Dene, Eastbourne Road and Branksome Terrace were areas of concern."

The film *A Clockwork Orange* (produced, adapted and directed by Stanley Kubrick) was released in 1972 and employed disturbing violent images to comment on psychiatry, juvenile delinquency, youth gangs and other social, political and economic subjects in a dystopian near-future Britain. It was controversial due to its depictions of graphic violence as well as, unfortunately, inspiring copycat acts of such violence that it was later withdrawn from British cinemas at Kubrick's behest.

Darlington even had its own Chapter of Hells Angels, based just off Duke Street, in the centre of town which most people kept away from. The gangs would come together, at football matches, and temporarily forget local animosities in order to focus collectively upon "out of towners" especially at games played against local rivals such as Hartlepool.

The 1970s, nationwide, was of course littered with hooliganism and especially when associated with football, deprivation, political unrest and lack of social amenities to occupy youths in the evenings and at the weekend.

If you are reading this you might be asking (as I would be) "this history is all fine and dandy but how does it lead to life as *A Patient Pharmacist*?"

The answer, of course is "It's ---- -- --- ---------."

Chapter 3

It's Just in the Chemistry

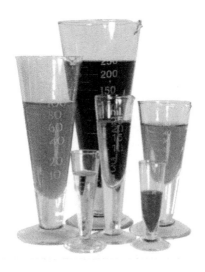

At school my brother and I showed a particular affinity for Chemistry and its experimentation which developed both into a risky hobby and professional careers. Mine organically as a pharmacist and his inorganically as a metallurgist (pun intended).

Our hobby evolved from filtration and growing crystal gardens to making home-made fireworks. The latter of which would today, I'm sure, have us on some "watch" list.

Together with my brother and his mate (both three years my elders, that's my get out clause) we went on a shopping list of ingredients from the local Chemist's shop.

Items included saltpetre (potassium nitrate) sold as fertiliser and in fact as a preservative (used in pate) but also marvellous oxidiser for rockets and fireworks, sulphur (used as an antibacterial for acne) to act as a fuel and to reduce ignition temperature to increase burn rate, sodium chlorate (weed killer), and iron filings to produce gold sparks. The acquisitions were appropriately mixed and packed into "humbug" tins, fuses were made using a solution from the mixture and the whole projectile placed in a cardboard tube as a launcher. We sloped off to the local woods and then Bang! our careers launched. My brother's mate later became a Submarine Commander! My brother was a metallurgist at a local steelworks, later becoming a policeman!

*

I don't exactly remember when my epiphany to be a pharmacist exactly occurred, yet I'm certainly sure (at the tender age of 12/13) it followed my firework shopping and visits to the local "Chemist" with my mam to collect some medicine and seeing the Chemist in a brilliant white lab coat, standing with a conical measure containing a blue liquid, high in the air, checking the correct levels. It was like a scene from Disney's *The Sorcerer's Apprentice* and I was hooked and transfixed as to what processes went on behind the counter.

Consequently, I kept my head down and "stuck in" at school to get my GCEs in order to attend Darlington Sixth Form College and take the relevant A levels required. Fortunately Chemistry, Biology (particularly Human Biology) and Maths were my favourite and most successful subjects and just the prescription for a Pharmacy course at University.

What was it about 1973 that made it so memorable for me?

Was it the fact that England joined the EEC (along with Denmark and Ireland)?

Was it that Sunderland beat the mighty, dominant Leeds United (by a single goal) in the 92nd FA Cup Final?

Was it the fact that at Bell Labs, New Jersey, the first cell phone call was made (The first mobile phone call was made 40 years ago today – The Atlantic) and Ethernet and fibre optics were created which massively changed the world and led to the mobile smartphone being the dominant technology today?

No, September 1973 was a pivotal and life-changing time for me. My friend's parents went to Blackpool for the weekend and, as teenagers are apt to do, my friend organised a party at his house. It was here that Carol and I (both aged 15) became an item (I was in love! It must have been the Chemistry again).

Carol was already in my class at Longfield Comprehensive School and I was the swot (her words) at the front of the class, but in reality I sat there because I needed glasses so had to sit at the front in order to read the board. She was the chatty one (my words) at the back with a bunch of her friends. A reversal of the musical *Grease*.

Perhaps it was the formula of opposites attract: both in a dress and music sense. Carol with her Crombie, two-tone "Staprest" trousers and creepers (love of Tamla Motown and to some degree Northern soul, but ultimately soul music) and me with my long hair, RAF blue grey trench coat, loon bell-bottomed jeans, platform shoes (love of heavy rock music including the likes of Deep Purple, Black Sabbath and Status Quo).

Or it was perhaps that we were both rebellious in our own ways (according to our parents, but I guess most parents say that of their teenage offspring). We also both had a love of sport (dance included for Carol, another opposite for me).

The only music we could agree to like and to listen to together was Simon and Garfunkel's *Bridge over troubled water* and Mike Oldfield's *Tubular Bells* (released that year). The first album I bought Carol was *Stevie Wonder's Greatest Hits* (1968 release which included such tracks as "Place in the Sun", "Fingertips Pt 2" and "Castles in the sand").

This was contrasted by Carol's gift to me of Black Sabbath's first album simply titled, *Black Sabbath* (including the tracks "The Wizard", "Evil Woman" and "Black Sabbath").

To this day we still buy each other an album/CD for Christmas.

As I have already said, I had a driven desire to become a pharmacist. My parents wanted me to be a doctor and go to Oxford/Cambridge but I was sticking to my guns.

I remember introducing Carol to my parents for the first time, in her words a moment of extreme trepidation.

A few days later, my dad took me to one side and to my dismay said to me, "Don't get too involved with a girl and throw your career away!" No doubt it was with the best intentions (in his eyes) but it incensed me and made me more determined than ever to follow my dreams of Pharmacy and being with the love of my life. We are 41 years and counting happily married.

Whilst at Sixth Form the careers tutor asked me which career I wanted to pursue and when I indicated Pharmacy, he told me that he would have a word with his friend who was the manager of the larger Boots store in Darlington.

So off I popped for an interview. I'm not so sure whether it was my charisma, career aspiration, my love for photography, the friendly word or all the above that led to me getting a Saturday job there.

That was 1974 and I pursued a career with Boots until 2003 (more of that later).

It then came to the time to fill in my UCAS application form and decide which university to go to, my choices were:

- Joint first – Bradford/Nottingham
- Second – Aston Birmingham
- Third – Manchester
- Last – Bath

The order you put them on the form was at the time both influential and controversial. I still feel trepidation for the students of today.

This was followed by visits and interviews and then the provisional offers which (in old money where A was an A, there were no stars) were as follows:

- Bradford C, D, D
- Nottingham C, C, C
- Aston C, C, D
- Manchester no offer for Pharmacy but D, D, E for Botany!
- Bath no offer (I guess they didn't take kindly to being put last)

So the next step was, of course, to sit the exams. And await the results. Only a few distractions to my studies, namely my love of table football (a.k.a. Foosball).

The Darlington Queen Elizabeth Sixth Form College was a stand-alone unit (all schools in Darlington didn't have a sixth form) which was an excellent precursor to University in that there was no uniform and it had a brilliant common room where you were able to feel like adults (in theory at least).

In this common room there was a juke box (which incessantly played Minnie Ripperton's "Loving You") but more importantly a table football table. Every spare hour (and many not so) was played on this. I used to arrive early each day and play for 30 minutes, at least before first lessons, during break times and often in General Studies lesson time which we were often dragooned back into by teachers. (We were encouraged to take General Studies lessons but did not have to take the A level, a "grounding" exercise no doubt.)

This affection for table football continued throughout University and as such I felt reasonably proficient at it (proportionally representative of time and resource put in, like most of life in general).

It was around this time (aged 17) that I passed my motorbike test on my beloved Yamaha 80cc 2 stroke street bike. This enabled me to pillion passenger Carol to Darlington Technical College on my way to Sixth Form (Aww, I hear you say). Previously, I used to travel on the Darlington Corporation buses to Carol's house and to College.

Carol used to live at Bloomfield Road in the Denes area of Darlington (formed in its North West area by the Pease family in the 1860s) and I used to live at North Road, Harrowgate Hill (North East area in the Whessoe Parish, named after Whessoe, a metal engineering firm, founded in 1790 and formerly supplying chemical, oil and nuclear plant instrumentation). There was no direct link East to West, which meant catching one bus into the centre of Darlington and then another up Woodland Road to Tower Road followed by a short walk to Bloomfield Road.

This walk up Tower Road was a little "spooky" on a dark night as it took you past a clock tower, out buildings and a synagogue which appeared very gothic indeed (straight out of a Hammer House of Horror movie) and could set your mind racing and imagining visions of ghosts, vampires and werewolves, the hooting owls and occasional bats also added to the atmosphere. I was so delighted, then, to have my own transport to avoid this.

Like all students, I waited with great anxiety for my results (as I thought I'd failed some, a feeling in common over all generations no doubt).

Anyhow the letter box rattles and a pre-stamped and addressed envelope plops onto the carpet. Inside of which is a slip of paper with the simple words:

- A level Mathematics with Statistics – Grade B
- A Level Chemistry – Grade B
- A Level Biology – Grade A

I'm not sure who was shocked the most, me or my parents. It was now time to choose and Bradford was my choice. Why? I'll let you decide!

Could it be because:

- Bradford has been teaching Pharmacy since 1927 and offered a three or four year undergraduate Bachelor of Pharmacy (with Honours)
- It was in Yorkshire and I'm a Yorkshireman (Middlesbrough born)
- It was far enough away from home
- My brother was attending Sheffield Polytechnic for his metallurgy degree
- My aunt and uncle and nanna lived in Mirfield, close by
- Carol was going to Hull College to study for a teaching degree and Hull has close rail links with Bradford

So it was off to Bradford with both trepidation and excitement like many a Fresher.

But, before me going to Bradford and Carol going to Hull we decided to take a holiday together, it was the summer of '76 after all. We had watched an episode of

Holiday '76 on BBC1 about "Skewjack" surf village in Cornwall and we were hooked, and so decided to book a week's holiday learning to surf. Our parents were old fashioned (how different it was back then to these modern times) and so we told them that our accommodation was in single sex dormitories but in actual fact it was a chalet with a double bed! Crazy it must sound as we were 18 but respected our parents' views. Bags were packed, with all the appropriate beach gear vital for such a hot summer, and we caught the Friday 8pm train from York all the way through to Penzance, arriving at 6am Saturday morning.

What an overnight journey, it was the Royal Mail train which stopped at almost every city station along the way dropping off and picking up mail and parcels. The carriages were of the compartment type with two bench seats facing each other, which could each accommodate four people, with a wooden sliding door separating the corridor which connected the other carriage compartments. Fortunately for 90% of the journey we had the compartment to ourselves and so could lounge out on the seats and "cuddle up" through the night which was so cold because the compartment's heating did not operate and we had not packed any warm clothes. An abiding memory of this journey was a guard, around 5am. walking down the corridor shouting, in a deep Cornish accent, "Next stop Redruth". We still joke about it whenever we visit Cornwall.

When we arrived at 6am, at Penzance station, only the café beside the taxi rank and harbour was open but at least we could get a much needed bacon butty and a hot drink, We then had another six hours to kill before our transport arrived to take us to the surf village and so we kept wandering around the town centre and harbour visiting more coffee bars once open.

At around mid-day "Amy", an old ambulance, arrived (which would become our daily transport for the whole holiday taking us and our surf boards to west Cornwall's beaches of Sennen Cove, Gwenever and Porthcurno) to take us to the surf village.

Skewjack Surf Village was located about 1.5 miles east of Land's End at the site of RAF Sennen whose buildings were converted into chalet accommodation by Chris Tyler and was to become the forerunner of surfing camps and surf schools in the UK, Europe and the world.

Facilities on site included a shop, bistro, bar, disco and pool and the holiday price included use of wetsuits, surfboards, tuition and transport. On top of all this there were beach football matches, softball, skateboarding, table tennis, darts tournaments, barbeques, midnight movies, bicycle hire, fancy dress and loony evenings and Thursday evening Magical Mystery Tours.

Entertainment was devised for each night of the week including disco nights, medieval banquets and pub crawls by boat to the fishing port of Newlyn and the villages of Mousehole and Lamorna Cove. The surfing was great but always followed by drinking in the pub or the on-site "Sunset Bar" which served ice cold lagers and beers and the infamous Harvey Wallbanger cocktail.

Songs played at the disco which to this day revive our memories of this week include "Don't go breaking my heart" by Elton John and Kiki Dee, "Let 'em in" by Billy Paul, "Save your kisses for me" by Brotherhood of Man, "Misssissippi" by Pussycat, "Living next door to Alice" by Smokie and of course "Mamma Mia" and "Fernando" by Abba.

It was a "scorching" week weather wise and, despite our sunburn and partying we managed some success with the longboards (by day five I was able to remain standing as I surfed) and avoided broken limbs, but the same couldn't be said for all guests as there were several broken arms and legs as people nosedived off the front of the board and were subsequently pounded by the surf into the sloping beach.

Carol and I did manage one night off to have a romantic meal at the Tin Mine Tavern, near St Just, reached by taxi.

What an adventure for 18-year-olds to prepare us for what was to come at University.

*

It was at Bradford, whilst in Halls of Residence and sharing some less than salubrious student houses, (to put it mildly) that I met and still retained many friends from all parts of the country each doing different and varying degrees (from Social Sciences, Manufacturing Systems Engineering, Geography through to Economics etc.) A "right" mix of characters.

We still (at least annually) get together in order to reminisce, chew the fat and "take the Mickey" out of each other, just as we did some 45 years ago. We even have a WhatsApp group (appropriately titled "Bradford") where we daily "chat" about issues of the day. Just Like Grumpy Old Men.

There are lots of tales (similar to many students in many places) to be told of those years, but I believe that is better suited to a different book (perhaps collaboratively with better writers than myself).

It can be said that the time between 1976 and 1979 at Bradford University was challenging both educationally and socially.

1978–9 was described as "The Winter of Discontent" there were freezing conditions (not conducive to learning or the impoverished student pocket in order to stay warm) and mass strikes.

The strikes started with Ford workers with subsequent

public sector workers also striking. Binmen, nurses, train drivers, lorry drivers and even gravediggers withdrew their labour.

76–79 were also years in which Bradford saw National Front demonstrations and violent racist attacks against Asian Britons. The NF saw Bradford as a fertile recruiting ground and also saw students as empathetic to Asians (which of course we were) and so would attack us if we were isolated. This led to "not going in" to the central city area of Bradford on weekend evenings unless in significant groups. (Fortunately a large group of my friends played rugby for the university and so felt safer but very wary and vulnerable at the same time.)

1975–1980 was also the murderous period of Peter Sutcliffe "The Yorkshire Ripper" several of whose atrocious and violent murders happened in Bradford (and in some cases in streets nearby to the student houses we lived in). This period of time created an atmosphere of fear amongst women in the Leeds/Bradford and indeed whole of the West Yorkshire areas. During this time we all always ensured that our girlfriends, housemates, fellow female students and colleagues were accompanied around the city.

As some of the murders happened so locally many students such as myself were interviewed by West Yorkshire Police on several occasions as part of their wide ranging investigations. Some idiot sent a "tape" to the police purporting to be "The Ripper" with a North Eastern accent which led to those of us from the NE receiving more questioning.

However, my time at Bradford University was indeed very happy and despite partying and at least fortnightly weekend visits to Hull College, I achieved my degree.

I had managed to get a "Desmond" (named after Desmond Tutu the South African Anglican bishop). That is a 2:2 Bachelor of Pharmacy (with honours) degree that was presented by Harold Wilson (former Prime Minister and Chancellor of the University of Bradford).

The degree course covered a broad range of related topics, leading to many employment opportunities such as pharmaceutical manufacturing and research, academia, hospital or retail pharmacy. It was upon the latter path I followed.

The topics that would help me along the way included such confusing sounding names as:

Pharmacy Law and Ethics essential to operate and practise legally as a registered pharmacist. Notable and essential Acts to know and follow were the *Pharmacy and Poisons Act 1933* (even drugs for human use were known and regulated as poisons), the *Medicines Act 1968* (still in force today and classified medicines under three categories POM, P and GSL) and finally the *Misuse of Drugs Act 1971* (which made possession of listed drugs an offence without a prescription and supply and storage of both strictly enforced and regulated). More on storage in the cabinet with the "golden key" later.

These lectures were probably the most boring (delivered in a 120 seater lecture theatre from a lecturer using a scrolling overhead projector at a "rate of knots") but, probably, the most important and essential to a Retail Pharmacist.

Biopharmaceutics defined as "the study of the physical and chemical properties of drugs and their proper dosage as related to the onset, duration, and intensity of drug action". This has become more essential to the pharmacist role as it is continually evolving into a much needed clinical support role in today's NHS. As is:

Clinical Pharmacology defined gloriously as "that discipline that teaches, does research, frames policy, gives information and advice about the actions and proper uses of medicines in humans and implements that knowledge in clinical practice".

This topic was delivered both in lecture and practical experimental forms. In one notable set of experiments we had to (under strict medical supervision) take certain medicines and measure their physiological effects upon ourselves. I particularly remember the experiment in which we were each given different types of diuretic (water tablets) and told to measure its effects on urine volume and frequency. Unknown (a blind experiment) to me I was given the powerful furosemide. I was "peeing" for Britain and having to dash rapidly and frequently to the loo with my large volume measure. An experiment which inevitably led to my empathy for anyone who is prescribed said diuretics.

Other experiments included taking different sedative drugs (including antihistamines, barbiturates, anti-anxiety drugs) and measuring their effects on cognitive function and EEG (brain activity) tracing.

Asthma and other drugs to help breathing were tried which involved wearing a backpack (to collect expired air) a lot of running up and down stairs and exercise bike pedalling, spirometer tubes and wires all designed to measure lung function.

Some drugs which affect heart function such as beta blockers were also tested along with blood pressure, heart rate monitoring together with ECG (heart) tracing.

Memorable experiments all, but little did I know at this time of being an experimental guinea pig, that later in my life they would become essential diagnostics in my health treatment, namely cognitive function (pharmacy register retention) heart function (suspected heart attack) brain function (epilepsy and brain tumour) of which more will be explained later.

Physiology simply "the study of how the human body

works".

Microbiology (including, virology, bacteriology, immunology, mycology and parasitology) the "scientific study of microorganisms." This involved growing cultures and their microscopic examination using aseptic (sterile) techniques.

Pharmaceutical Chemistry which built upon my earlier firework experimentation. Very practical based which also involved many experiments to identify a drug or chemical compounds by burning, melting, distilling, filtering, centrifuging, dissolving in various liquids, spectrometry and gas chromatography. An alchemist's arsenal.

Pharmacognosy defined as the "study of medicines or crude drugs produced from natural sources such as plants, microbes, and animals". This involved many an hour looking down the microscope at plant structures, not my favourite subject (reference back to Botany degree offer). However, plants of course throughout history have formed the basis of many medicines.

The word Trichome (a fine appendage on plants) springs to mind as I remember this study, it also reminds me of a little ditty penned for an end of year review.

It is in the tune and style of Tom Jones's "Green, Green Grass of Home" and was as follows

"Down the lens I look,
And there's a Trichome
I couldn't tell if it was
A tree or dog bone
Oh the green green plants of home"
Such was my love of plants.

Dispensing Techniques this references the "Sorcerer's Apprentice" earlier and utilises and teaches use of all the equipment in the apothecary's arsenal. Essential to my early years as a Pharmacist, it was here that I learnt to use the mortar and pestle, various weighing balances, conical measures, ointment slabs, pessary moulds, powder folders. Also, I learnt how to follow formulas to make mixtures, ointments, creams, lotions and potions, powders, pills, cachets, infusions, injections, enemas and suppositories etc.

I am sure there were other topics as well, but now not so easily remembered.

Chapter 4

Supplementing my Grant (Work)

As aforesaid, I had a Saturday job at Boots prior to University and this paid dividends in that as a Pharmacy student I was able to work all holidays throughout my studies at their Darlington branch. Not only did this provide much needed funding for holidays, clothing, an engagement ring and socialising but also served as a valuable career influence and experience.

This would initially be work on the photographic counter (Chemists and Druggists have had a long association with the supply of photographic equipment and chemicals), progressing to the "Chemist Counter" and then finally the holy grail "The Dispensary".

Boots had excellent in-store training (aided by external suppliers) and I attended most relevant and available courses. This included such topics as photography skills, camera equipment product knowledge, watch battery replacement, battery knowledge and even Homebrew (wine and beer making) skills.

Life on the photographic counter involved "taking in" films for processing (hoping that the processors didn't lose any precious memories). Many an hour was spent in the dark with my hands stuffed into a lightproof camera bag to rescue films which had snapped or stuck in the myriad of different cameras available. I sold many different brands (Kodak, Polaroid, Agfa, Fuji and Boots Own Brand) and types (35mm, 126, 110, cartridge, 127, 120, 620 roll, instant picture, Black and White and Slide) of film. But perhaps the most successful, in sales terms (particularly at Christmas and New Year), was "The Magicube".

The "Magicube" was a cheap flash for 1970s cameras which in order to produce its flash was like having a small piece of explosive confined within a glass bulb surrounded by a protective plastic cube (four explosion flashes per cube). Back to my firework and gunpowder days.

Why battery knowledge and watch battery training you could ask? Firstly, batteries were one of the most profitable items sold and secondly in 1975 Sinclair launched its "Black Watch", an innovation ahead of its time though it later became a commercial disaster. The watch had a red LED display, which only became visible when one part of the outer case was pressed thereby displaying hours and minutes and then pressing another part displayed minutes and seconds.

This watch had technical problems with its integrated circuit and short battery life. The batteries only had an actual ten day life (despite advertising claiming a year) as well as being very difficult to replace.

Scientific programmable calculators became a key (pun) sales item with the likes of the Sinclair Scientific Programmable being introduced into the UK in August 1975 costing £49.95 (equivalent to £500+ at 2022 levels). An invaluable instrument to many a student such as me.

Other brands sold included those by Hewlett-Packard, Texas Instruments and Casio.

The photographic counter was next to the record counter and I would often stray onto the latter (such was my love of music). Two memories of this spring to mind. One was that on a particular day (16th August 1977) Delta (anonymised name) the Supervisor started crying and shrieking "The King is Dead" obviously meaning Elvis Presley.

The second was the shop's "store detective" screaming, "Help Help" as he was chasing an individual with about 20 LP music albums (at the time such items were out on "live display") tucked under their coat out the side door. So off I "legged it" after them managing (only with reasonable and necessary force) to grab hold of the suspected shoplifter. However, the said individual produced a "shiny sharp-looking object" from their coat which caused me to rapidly release them. No way was I going to be injured in the line of duty. They were later apprehended by police and a further 20 LPs recovered from behind a wall. This was not the only (by a long way) shoplifting incident that I had to deal with over my career.

Time served on the photo counter led me to the chemist counter and the more and more I progressed through University with some Pharmacy knowledge gained (or so I thought) the more and more it became my workplace.

At first it seemed daunting thinking that I might be asked about, and for, things that I had little or no knowledge of but at least I had the support of experienced staff.

I was very young and was not cherishing people asking me about "condoms". In those days they were mainly obtained at places such as the barbers when asked, "Would you like something for the weekend, sir?" Or you would buy them surreptitiously while buying something else when you thought nobody was paying attention.

Anyway I was bewildered by this American individual (not the last time either) who came up to me and boomed the words "Where are the prophylactics, mate?" I just stood frozen.

With my limited Pharmacy education I thought that they wanted a particular type of medicine to prevent a disease condition. A member of staff eased my embarrassment by telling me that in North America a prophylactic meant condom! They also told me that a few years back Boots had only sold them under the counter and then in paper bags. A little known fact is that up until the 1960s Boots would not sell condoms at all lest it encourage promiscuity, and even after 1961 staff were reminded that the only exception was "where they are ordered by a medical man himself, or where a genuine prescription is handed in". Lord Trent, son of Boots' founding father, asked his co- directors, "Would you like to see your daughters selling these things?"

Thank goodness times changed rapidly, correctly and effectively from this early stance.

Anyway time now leads me to my entry and first practical experience of "The Dispensary".

*

In the store "The Dispensary" was in a prominent location on a raised level (about three steps above the chemist counter level) with unrestricted views across the shop floor (even a good straight view to the photographic counter so I hadn't strayed far). It had a screen all round just like a castle battlements which you could see over but they could not clearly see in.

The public could of course see me holding up a glass conical measure checking liquid levels with a high degree of accuracy (I am now indeed "The Sorcerer's Apprentice").

One of my early tasks was just like working behind a bar in that the first job of the day was to stack the bottles shelves full (not with beer and pop bottles but with medicine bottles and jars). These medicines bottles came in all shapes and sizes, tablet bottles both round and square, liquid medicine bottles and brown ribbed glass bottles, the ribbing to indicate either an external use liniment or lotion or even a "poison".

At this stage I was also allowed to count tablets and put together pre-filled bottles containing some of the most commonly prescribed medicines of the time such as paracetamol (Panadol), diazepam (Valium) and Ibuprofen (Brufen) etc. Brufen was discovered in 1961 by two (Adams and Nicholson) Boots UK Ltd employees and first marketed in the UK in 1969 and then in the USA in 1974.

Counting during this period of time was done predominately manually using a "Dispensing Triangle" i.e. no electronic counting machines nor robots, which are very much in use today.

This equilateral triangle, usually made from plastic or extruded aluminium, was an ingenious invention. Basically the method was to tip the tablets (any round, or hexagonal even size, convex, or concave) from the bulk container (of say 500, or 1000 tablets) onto the triangle and count the numbers of rows, settled after shaking the triangle to level the tablets flat and then to simply pour the required number into your correctly selected tablet bottle.

Rows	1	2	3	4	5	6	7	8	9
Tablets	1	3	6	10	15	21	28	36	45

Rows	10	11	12	13	14	15	16	17	18
Tablets	55	66	78	91	105	120	136	153	171

So simply if you wanted 100 tablets you chose either 13 rows and added a further nine tablets, or 14 rows taking five tablets away whichever was the quickest and you became the most adept at. Most tablets nowadays are packaged in foil strips and strips cut to match the number required.

Pharmacy during this time was still a technical skill requiring certain medicines, especially mixtures, lotions, and creams, still to be "made up" in the dispensary.

At this stage I was also allowed to make up pre-filled mixtures such as Magnesium Trisilicate (which involved three powders consisting of 5% each of magnesium trisilicate, light magnesium carbonate, and sodium bicarbonate in a suitable liquid vehicle with a peppermint flavour) which sold in significant amounts as a stomach antacid.

This involved practising using those skills learnt in my dispensing techniques element of my degree course. Namely using the mortar and pestle mechanical prescription balances and various measures.

When using the balances, in order for weight accuracy, you had to ensure that the spirit level on said balance was "dead centre". However, at my first attempt I thought that for speed that instead of putting the scale balance on the dispensing bench I could just weigh the very light bulky powders on the scales "in situ" on the shelf. (I had already checked that they were set "dead centre".)

But as I piled up the powders on the scale pan I knocked it and the whole set of scales, powders and weights crashed from a height to the floor and sent a plume of white powder into the air covering one and all in the dispensary just like a plume of ash from a volcano. Needless to say this did not "go down well" with the experienced staff. Fortunately no one was hurt and I was able to continue my work and practice.

Another task given was to complete the daily drug ordering over the telephone. For this I had to memorise the phonetic alphabet. This set of code words was accepted by NATO in 1956 with the intention of letters

(26) and numbers being easily distinguishable from one another over radio and telephone. Alpha for A Mike for M, Zulu for Z etc. I still recall and use it to this day.

All drug containers in the dispensary had a stock card attached. On the card top was a five digit code such as "PRO 10" and on the one side of the body of the card was the description such as "propranolol 10mg tablets quantity 500".

And on the other side the quantity and date ordered and how many needed to be kept in stock. So as you finished a bottle of said tablets you simply marked the card with the quantity to order and the date and then put the cards in A–Z order on a board. Each day you had a telephone time slot to place your order to the drug warehouse.

So in this example I would say "Papa Romeo Oscar ten by one" and hopefully the next day we would receive one 500 tablet container of Propranolol 10mg strength tablets.

A simple effective system replaced later of course by computer labelling systems ordering automatically.

During the '70s and early '80s medicines were mainly labelled with handwritten labels or partially typed with details pre-printed such as "Take ONE tablet THREE times a day" and the address of the Pharmacy (Chemist) onto which you then wrote the patient's name and any further instructions.

The name of the medication (and quantity) was also written unless the prescriber gave instruction (by annotation) that they did not want the name placed on the label in which case it was labelled as just "The Tablets" or "The Mixture" with a reference number. Sometimes this was for best intentions such as prescribing a placebo or complicated formula mixture for which the prescriber did not want the patient to worry about its contents such as for palliative pain relief.

Such a mixture was the "Brompton cocktail" (other names included Brompton Mixture, Mistura euphoriens, Mistura pro moribunda, Saunders' and Hoyle's mixture) which was first introduced in the BNF (British National Formula) in 1976. Its first origins date to 1952 at the Brompton Hospital under the name Haustus E (probably meaning draught elixir). The original formula being based as follows (with many later variations) and was used as an "on demand" pain relief in palliative care.

- Morphine hydrochloride ¼ grain
- Cocaine hydrochloride ⅙ grain
- Alcohol 90% 30 minims
- Syrup 60 minims
- Chloroform water to ½ fl. Oz.

One grain was a unit in the troy weight, avoirdupois, and Apothecaries' system, equal to exactly 64.79 milligrams. One Fluid Ounce (Imperial) is 480 minims. The formula was converted to metric for simplification but in the very early stage of my career we had measures in minims and weights in grains. Over the years the formula was also modified to substitute the alcohol 90% for whisky, brandy or vodka, whichever was the patient's preferred choice. Sometimes an anti-sickness (antiemetic) drug was also added.

Chapter 5

The Golden Key

Well not a key made from gold but rather brass which locked/unlocked the Controlled Drugs cabinet.

Under the "Misuse of drugs Act 1971" certain categories (schedules) of controlled drugs had to be stored in a specialised metal (steel) cabinet bolted and secured firmly in its dispensary location with the access key in the pharmacist's actual possession or under their personal control. Many such drugs including pharmaceutical grade powders (Diamorphine, Morphine and Cocaine), injection vials (Diamorphine, Cocaine, Pethidine and Dipipanone) and suppositories of the same as well as other forms and drugs.

Sometimes other substances were stored there as well, more of that later.

Over my many years as a pharmacist (and for many pharmacists of today) this control was always in the forefront of my mind as was the security and the correct legal supply of such powerful drugs.

All receipt and supply of any quantities of such drugs had to be recorded in the "Controlled Drugs Register" and records kept for the legal requisite amount of time and open for viewing and checks and balances by authorised officials (Pharmaceutical Society and The Home Office Inspectors as well as Drug Squad Officers).

All this talk of formula and key and register control is just background information for the next story.

Once having obtained the Bachelor of Pharmacy degree you were required to undertake a year's further training in a registered retail or hospital pharmacy under the direct supervision, assessment and mentoring of a pharmacist registered (by the Royal Pharmaceutical Society of Great Britain) to undertake pre-registration graduate training.

This I was fortunate to be able to do in the same Darlington store in which I worked during my vacations. This involved regular (three-monthly) assessments and reports sent to the RPSGB by the Pre-Registration Tutor Pharmacist and after 12 months the tutor sent a final report stating whether you were able and met the ethical, clinical and practical skills in order to be registered as a Pharmacist (nowadays the students also have to sit an RPSGB written examination test). In fact over my career I also was such a tutor, responsible for a dozen or so pharmacists achieving their registration status (a role not taken lightly and with great responsibility).

The whole year was also to practise all the skills learnt at university and some new "on the job" skills (such as hosiery and truss measurement and fitting).

One day I was in the dispensary with a locum pharmacist (from Sunderland wearing a green suit, it's strange what you remember whether relevant or not).

The said locum received a prescription for the "Brompton Cocktail", as discussed previously, and so being in possession of the "golden key" opened up the CD cabinet and took out the necessary ingredients (including brandy on this occasion). He then accurately weighed and measured the required quantities and recorded in the CD register what was used and supplied. The patient's relative then duly collected the bottle of mixture.

About 30 minutes later the locum began to sweat and became somewhat animated. "John, John," he shouted. "I've forgotten to put the cocaine in that patient's Brompton."

So he concocted a plan to solve this problem to ensure that the patient was able to get the appropriate amount of pain relief. It did, however, involve me acting as a "courier" much to my concern.

He then weighed the correct amount of cocaine powder, and then using paper, and a brass powder folder (which looked like a miniature deck chair with razor-sharp edges), folded the cocaine into a precise folded paper. This was an origami type skill learnt at University for drug powder dispensing (like a "Beechams' Powder" for those of you old enough to remember).

He then gave the "powder" to me and said, "John you go the patient's house straight away and then pour the powder into the patient's bottle. In the meanwhile I'll telephone them to say that you are on your way."

Of course I could not drive and so had to catch the "Corporation" bus. So here I was sat on the bus with a significant amount of 100% pure pharmaceutical grade cocaine in my pocket (scared stiff that I could be stopped by a policeman and having to try and explain why). This could have possibly led to me not being able to register as a pharmacist. However, I did have "insurance" in my other pocket in the form of a letter of explanation signed by said pharmacist on official headed paper with his contact details and Pharmaceutical Society registration number.

The theory of "Truss" fitting was simple enough but the practical application not so. The truss is a kind of surgical appliance used for patients with a hernia (which occurs when an internal part of the body pushes through a weakness in the muscle or surrounding tissue wall), providing support for the herniated area, using a pad and belt arrangement to hold it in the correct position. This herniation usually develops between your chest and lungs. Usually named as umbilical (abdominal), inguinal (hip area of groin) or scrotal (descending into the scrotal sac). The truss belt was made of elastic band webbing or cloth-covered spring steel with firm pads of various shapes and sizes.

As a student the measurement was practised on a clothed individual, by measuring the circumference around the hip at the ileac crest area (curved area at the top of the ilium bone, the largest of three bones that make up the pelvis).

However, in actual practise this was undertaken on a naked (waist down) patient. The truss had to be fitted next to the skin ensuring that the hernia swelling could be retracted into the cavity before fitting. You can probably imagine the first-time trepidation when you asked the patient to drop their undergarments and you were presented with swellings (hernias) of various shapes and sizes (I now realised why I didn't want to be a doctor). Currently most doctors and surgeons do not prescribe trusses, due to better surgery availability using improved techniques (such as endoscopy) and to prevent complications that the truss itself could cause. This was also a blessing when I became a patient requiring such intervention following (later described) surgical complications.

The other skill to be developed (during this pre-registration training year) was that of hosiery measuring and fitting. The hosiery that was prescribed (mainly to alleviate varicose veins by helping venous blood flow return by compression of the veins) was bulky and cumbersome and was either flat-bed knit (one-way stretch) or circular knit (two-way stretch).

Circumference measurements at various points along the thigh, knee, calf, ankle and foot were taken. The garment/s were then ordered and were specially made for that individual. Now these stockings had to be held up somehow so you can imagine the consternation of many a male patient when told they would need to wear a surgical suspender belt or suspender straps attached by buttons to each pair of trousers worn (a bit more palatable). I must admit most patients just took it in their stride and accepted their fate.

These fittings became extremely rare in my later career and much better hosiery is now available including TENS compression stockings which are tight-fitting stretchy socks that apply gentle pressure to feet and legs to help blood flow in the body. (I have many pairs following my many surgical operations.)

Chapter 6

Habenda Ratio Valetudinis

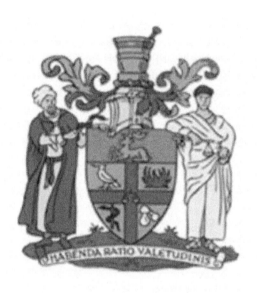

So it was, in July 1980, that I became a registered Member of the Royal Pharmaceutical Society of Great Britain (MRPharmS.) That is a fully qualified pharmacist (and official golden key holder) and able to operate as such.

"Habenda ratio valetudinis" is the Society motto and its meaning is, "A means of good health is requiring to be had" or "Account must be taken of health".

It is with this in "mind" that I functioned as a working pharmacist and as a patient too.

My first support role was to cover holidays and days

off for Boots branch (store) pharmacists in my local area.

My patch was the lovely Yorkshire and Durham Dales area and included such towns as Darlington (of course), Richmond, Ripon, Thirsk, Northallerton, Knaresborough and Barnard Castle.

Barnard Castle is of course an ancient historic town in its own right but has recently been further "put on the map" by the infamous visit of the Prime Minister's (Boris Johnson) Chief Adviser, Dominic Cummings. It is reputed that during the Covid 19 lockdown and pandemic that he fled London to stay in a more remote family location (his parents' farm) in Durham. Before returning to London, it was said that in order to check problems with his eyesight he took a detour to "Specsavers" in Barnard Castle and was then spotted walking beside the River Tees and the castle. I'm not political (I leave that commentary for the better qualified "Bradford" lads) and yet it is a lovely walk and I went there in my lunch hours to eat my butties and in fact have returned many times to Barnard Castle to stay at the Motorhome and Caravan club site and still do to this day.

Barnard Castle is a traditional market town and people from all over the Wear and Tees valleys trip in particularly on market days. This local Boots branch (which used to have a farms and gardens annex at the rear) could be very busy at times. On one visit with the "golden key" (passed to me like an Olympic baton) I opened the "CD cabinet" and found to my horror and dismay an old tin of cyanide! (Cymag sodium cyanide).

I then had to contact Head Office to arrange for appropriate collection and disposal of it by licenced contractors. Sodium cyanide releases hydrogen cyanide gas, a highly toxic chemical asphyxiant that interferes with body's ability to use oxygen and can be rapidly fatal.

It was sold as a poison to farmers (under "The Poisons Act" requiring signed requisitions from the Ministry of Agriculture and Fisheries) to kill rabbits and vermin. Unfortunately it was also used in salmon poaching (the poachers used to throw a quantity of Cymag into the river at a fast flowing part upstream of a pool holding salmon, the salmon will effectively be suffocated, will thrash about on the surface, and once dead could be easily scooped out of the river as they float downstream).

Fortunately from the early 1980s it was no longer supplied from pharmacies and was removed from sale (anywhere) and use only allowed and disposal of stocks completed by end of 2004.

Another "poison" in the cabinet was strychnine (which was regularly sold and supplied in the 1980s, for the killing of moles and rats again under strict regulatory legal conditions of the Poisons Act 1972).

The supply could only be given upon production of a "Ministry of Agriculture and Fisheries permit" to an authorised individual personally known to you. If you did not know them, then they had to produce a signed letter of introduction, signed by a local policeman known to you. All supply and receipt of such poisons had to be entered into the poisons register (together with details of all parties and permits) and records kept for the required number of years.

Strychnine is a strong poison, only a small amount is needed to produce severe effects in people and even death (the extent of poisoning depends on the amount and route of exposure and pre-disposing health). It prevents the proper operation of the chemical that controls nerve signals to the muscles. It prevents the muscles "off switch" from working correctly causing severe painful spasms (without loss of consciousness and causing excitability) and the muscles eventually tire and the person can't breathe.

Of course today's Pharmacy has changed and no such poisons are supplied.

*

My time as a "Relief Pharmacist" was interesting and enjoyable to say the least. I did however want to progress into store management (Boots Store Managers at that time were all pharmacists).

Around November 1980 I received a telephone call from my "Territorial General Manager" asking me if I would like to transfer to Ipswich!

"Ipswich" I said "where is that?" I knew of the football team but not its geographical location. Apparently there was a shortage of pharmacists in Suffolk and the North East had a surplus (due to School of Pharmacy locations). So it was time to consult my bride to be, Carol.

I have previously hinted that my vocational employment was for funding an engagement ring, and on September 4th 1977 Carol and I officially got engaged (I had already popped the question from a phone booth in the Halls of Residence) and went for a meal at the Binchester Hall Hotel.

Binchester is another historical location of Roman significance (near Bishop Auckland) with the hotel on the grounds previously occupied by a Roman fort. Binchester Hall's history is linked with the Bowes-Lyon family, William van Mildert (Bishop of Durham) and branches of the Wren family (indeed Sir Christopher Wren is said to have designed the hall for the Durham branch of the Wrens, nestling it close to the Roman fort and perching it beside a delightful terrace, commanding a view of the picturesque vale of the Wear.)

A romantic location (at least so I thought) as in the 1960s it became a two star hotel with an 80 seat restaurant and its cellar bar was renowned as a nightclub, but then in the 1980s it became a nursing home (a theme that has more to run in my story).

Back to the wedding, which was scheduled for 11th July 1981, and so I needed Carol's thoughts and agreement that once married that we would move to Ipswich. Carol was at the time working as a Laboratory Technician at Longfield School which we had attended as pupils (despite qualifying as a teacher with a Bachelor of Education from Hull College, she could not get a teaching job) and would need to leave to join me in Ipswich. So in January 1981 off I went to work in Ipswich at its branch in Tavern Street. The upstairs stockroom here had wall to wall mirrors and oak panelling and was once a library.

Boots, at the instigation of Florence Boot, had a "Boots Book-lovers Library" in its stores from 1898 until 1966 (when it closed due to the "Public Libraries and Museums Act 1964" which required councils to provide free public libraries). Boots library was a subscription service.

From January, I worked in this branch as Supervising Pharmacist deputising for the Branch (store) Manager, living in hotel accommodation (only travelling home on alternate weekends, such is retail). This did exempt me from some of the minutiae of wedding planning but I did have to find a suitable home for us. Carol joined me, on occasion, for the shortlist approval.

*

We got married at South Cowton Church (North Yorkshire) attended of course by friends and family and some of the "Bradford" lads. Our wedding reception was at "The Terrace House Hotel" Richmond (North Yorkshire) which is now a nursing home!

So after our honeymoon (Yugoslavia) Carol and I

moved into our first home in Ipswich and I then again was "sent out" into "Relief Store Management" to cover for managers' holidays across Suffolk and Essex.

I remember the first time that I arrived at Ipswich station where a sign read "Harwich for the continent" (as you changed trains at Ipswich for the ferry at Harwich) and some bright spark had added the graffiti "Frinton for the Incontinent".

The branches worked included Frinton-on-Sea, Harwich, Clacton-on Sea, Walton-on-the-Naze, Colchester, Ipswich, Woodbridge, Felixstowe, Lowestoft, Stowmarket, Braintree, Witham, Southend-on-Sea, Bury St Edmunds, Saffron Walden and Chelmsford. All in all very much different to the North Yorkshire dales.

Ipswich and Suffolk possessed a collection of air force bases (both RAF and USA) including Bentwaters, Woodbridge and Mildenhall and their corresponding personnel covering many a nationality.

On one such occasion I was working at Woodbridge when this bold brash American strolled up to the counter and loudly asked, "Hey have you got anything for an itchy fanny?" I was still a little naïve at this stage (and of course knew they didn't mean a Japanese motorbike) and had to think on my feet, once I had gotten over the initial shock. I then asked the usual questions about who it was for, how long had they had the problem, any other symptoms, had they tried any medication and were they taking any current medication? From their response the penny soon dropped that "fanny" in the USA did not have the same meaning as in the UK. For the uninitiated, in the USA it refers to the rectum (hence the expression fanny bag for a bum bag) and in the UK it refers to the vagina. As such I was then able to recommend the appropriate remedy which hopefully was a cure.

On one particular Saturday morning I found myself in

charge of the Felixstowe branch (Felixstowe was, and still is, a major UK port, being the UK's largest container port and also used to operate as a ferry terminal to Zeebrugge, Belgium) when I received a telephone call from "Her Majesty's Customs and Excise" team based at the port. They had arrested a foot passenger trying to smuggle cannabis resin into the UK by strapping blocks around their body under clothing. (This is reminiscent of the 1978 film *Midnight Express*, a true crime drama about Billy, an American caught smuggling hashish in Turkey.) The reason for their call was that before the suspect could be charged and detained they needed an accurate weight of the said resin and as the local government Assay Office was closed could they bring it to me for weighing.

So it was that two officers in black suits (like a scene from *Men in Black*) one carrying two suitcases handcuffed to each wrist and the other just looking menacing appeared. ID cards were shown and I led them to the manager's office at the rear of the store where I had set up the manual beam weighing balances (Class A and Class B).

All pharmacies had to have accurate scales and weights which were inspected and tested on a regular basis by both the "Weights and Measures" and the "RPSGB" inspectorates. We also had a quarterly service schedule with "Avery" the manufacturers.

Now the issue with the office was that it did not have any windows and it was a very hot sunny day in Sleepy Suffolk. The large resin blocks (of which there were 24) began to sweat (as did we) and by the time the job was complete I'm convinced we were all "high" and needed some time, fresh air and a cup of tea to recover. It was during this chat time that they anecdotally described an arrest concerning a Rolls Royce suspiciously parked on the promenade in Frinton-on-Sea, which on further forensic examination revealed bags of heroin compacted into each of its large tyres an absolute fortune's worth on the black market and a huge coup for Customs. Such was the lengths that drug dealers would go to.

Once the blocks had been weighed I recorded the individual weights (of each piece of evidence) on official "Boots" headed notepaper, signed and dated together with my qualifications and RPSGB registration number then wished the "Men in Black" on their way.

I had noticed that the further South I worked, the more we were presented with "private" rather than NHS prescriptions not just from local GP and veterinary practices but also from as "far afield" as Harley Street (London). The authenticity of such prescriptions needed close scrutiny for legality as they were often written on headed notepaper, A4 foolscap, notepad scraps and even vellum (Harley Street) some with copper plate fountain pen and pristine neat writing and some barely legible scrawled biro. These prescriptions needed "pricing up" to charge an appropriate fee to cover ingredient, compounding, container, overheads and "time taken" costs. There was loose guidance costings from the "Company" and RPSGB but inevitably you could within reason charge what you liked. However, all such prescriptions had to be recorded in a "prescription register" and details kept (for inspection) for the required number of years.

It was once again in the holiday resort of Felixstowe where I was presented with an unusual veterinary private prescription. The circus had come to town and its lion "Leo" (an original name I know but true) had a fungal toenail infection and an antifungal cream was ordered to a specific formula which had to be made in the dispensary. So I counted the appropriate quantity of antifungal tablets and crushed them up in a mortar and pestle to produce a powder. The appropriate amount of a base cream was also selected and weighed. Then out came the large glass "ointment" slab and spatulas. The powder was then evenly dispersed using what's called a trituration technique. This involved placing a small amount of the powder and an equal amount of cream and spreading it across the slab (much in the same way that a plasterer plasters a wall). This was repeated and repeated "doubling up" the quantities each time until all the powder was evenly dispersed throughout all the cream and then put into a large jar. The jar labelled as follows:

"The Cream
To be applied Twice a day to the affected nail
FOR ANIMAL TEATMENT ONLY
FOR EXTERNAL USE ONLY
Leo the Lion C/O Chipperfields' Circus Felixstowe"

I had a vision of "Daniel" being thrown into the lions' den and wondered how the keeper would manage to apply it.

So it was that I had a great experience travelling around Suffolk and Essex. It was due to all these travels that I began to have an appreciation of the beauty of the area. In fact we regularly had friends and family come to visit for a "holiday" and I would don my hat and act as a tourist guide.

I remember taking our parents for an idyllic rowing boat excursion on the river Stour at Dedham to view the beautiful "Constable" countryside and Flatford Mill (The Haywain). Just as we were meandering slowly along up popped (literally) a group of completely naked men and women in all their morning glory. The looks on my mother's and mother-in-law's face were an absolute picture. So wild swimming is not a recent phenomenon.

When we first moved to Ipswich, as we did not know anyone, Carol and I decided to participate in a sport in which we could take part together. So we chose volleyball (which incidentally was popular in and around Ipswich especially with the American service men and women).

Volleyball has been such a great team sport for us from which we also made many a long lasting friendship. (Carol played for Ipswich and then Tamworth ladies teams and I have played for teams across the country.) We both played in leagues on a very competitive but also very social basis.

It was also on one of these nights that we were invited to a party in a house adjoining Bobby Robson's and were allowed access to Bobby's outdoor swimming pool and sauna.

Ipswich in 1981–82 had an excellent football team and Carol and I used to go and watch all their home fixtures. Portman Road was such a friendly ground and we stood on the terraces enthralled (Carol stood on a milk crate for a better view). On the 6th May 1981 we had the absolute pleasure to watch the first leg of the UEFA Cup Final between Ipswich and AZ Alkmaar ('67). Ipswich won this leg 3–0 with goals by John Wark, Frans Thijssen and Paul Mariner. The second leg, in Holland, resulted in a 4–2 win to AZ which meant that Ipswich had won the UEFA Cup Final 5–4 on aggregate. What a team and triumph, managed by the late and great Sir Bobby Robson and including other brilliant players such as Paul Cooper, Terry Butcher, Mick Mills, Russell Osman, George Burley, Kevin Beattie, Arnold Muhren, Alan Brazil and Eric Gates.

Other entertainment to be had on a glorious summer's evening was watching Ipswich Speedway team "The Witches" who won the British league Knockout Cup in 1981(in their 47th season in the top tier of speedway in the UK). For speedway enthusiasts, famous "Witches" riders at the time included Preben Eriksen, John Cook, Nigel Flatman and Kevin Jolly.

After volleyball training (and the bar) on a Friday we used to invite team members and friends round for a further tipple and some "supper". I remember (in Ipswich) one specific Friday evening 2nd April 1982 we decided to switch on the late news.

We were transfixed to watch Argentina's full scale invasion of the Falkland Islands. We thought how was "Margaret" (Thatcher) going to respond and would we get "called up" to help in the war. Fortunately it was all over by June 14th but not before Britain lost five ships and tragically 256 lives and Argentina lost its only cruiser and 750 lives. Such a waste.

Carol and I decided to have an addition to the family and so like many other couples before and subsequently we bought a dog from a farm near Halstead. She was a cross between a working border collie and a black Labrador. We named her "Elkie" (after the singer Elkie Brookes, whom we had seen live at Ipswich Gaumant Theatre). Brookes was also Carol's maiden name. The exact timing of this purchase is a bit vague (Carol states that we purchased Elkie to keep her company whilst I was away). I was on the company promotion list and a further management role beckoned.

Chapter 7

The Midlands

So around September 1983 I was promoted to Assistant Manager at the Tamworth branch, a role which was diverting me more into general retail store management. However, I did have a full-time pharmacist running the dispensary for me for whom I "covered" for tea, lunch breaks, days off and holidays and so I still had a pharmacist role (and part golden key possession). The overall store manager was a pharmacist also.

Tamworth, again, is a destination steeped in history with a castle and is a market town in Staffordshire (14 miles North East of Birmingham) and it borders with North Warwickshire. Tamworth was the principal centre of Royal power of the Anglo-Saxon Kingdom of Mercia during the eighth and ninth centuries. Its industries include logistics (central location), engineering, clothing, brick, tile and paper manufacture. Until 2001 one of its factories was Reliant, which produced the Reliant Robin (a three wheeler car of *Only Fools and Horses* fame) as well as the Reliant Scimitar (a sports car).

So it was that I travelled frequently from Ipswich to Tamworth until we found a new house. (I used to travel to work very early on a Monday morning, then home again on a Tuesday evening, as my day off was a Wednesday, returning back to work early on a Thursday morning and then back home on a Saturday evening, a pattern which was to feature regularly throughout my career in differing locations.)

During this time I had left Carol without the car but with "Elkie" to look after her.

Poor Carol had to cycle to her place of work across the opposite side of Ipswich, and there and back again at lunchtime to let "Elkie" out for exercise and "constitution". Carol, at this stage, was working as a mentor, trainer and tutor at Suffolk Triangle NACRO (National Association for Care and Rehabilitation for Offenders).

Whilst looking for a new house (and selling our Ipswich first home) I was accommodated in a small hotel in Tamworth. It was called the "Shruberries" and part of it included an Italian Restaurant "Armando's" that was run by two very friendly Italians. There was a real positive upside (for me at least) as I "munched" my way through the menu (seafood spaghetti, veal, bolognaise, steaks etc.). As a regular resident they would also ask me each morning if I wanted something different other than from the menu for dinner that evening. They were very sociable and, several evenings a week after they closed the restaurant, we used to go together for a game of snooker and a pint at the local snooker club then back for a "Grappa" nightcap.

Tamworth at the time was described as a "Birmingham overspill" housing area and the newer modernist housing stock reflected this. As such we searched for our new home further afield, in easy commuting (by car) distance and so we alighted in the beautiful village of Austrey (seven miles North West of Tamworth and in North Warwickshire), whose parish in Saxon times belonged to the Mercian nobleman Wulfric.

Austrey had the essential local amenities such as a pub, "The Bird in Hand" and a church (not so essential for me) as well as a village shop.

Carol used to drive me to work and then she commuted onward to her place of work in South Birmingham for NACRO (she, fortunately, had managed to secure a transfer from Suffolk Triangle). When I needed the car she was able to commute by train from Tamworth (more of that doggy tale to follow).

As already intimated, my work role was changing and I was very much becoming more involved in store operations including stock replenishment, staff training (pharmacy and non-pharmacy staff), merchandising, marketing (including window dressing) and team leadership. I was still involved with the photographic (though now with a film processing minilab) counter and record and gardening department. I mention the windows purely because we had a large number of windows whose displays (which acted as promotion and retail theatre) had to be dressed regularly (with a clear themed focus) by my full-time window dresser. The dressed windows were not quite like Harrods (London) nor Fenwicks (Newcastle) but more like the comparison of Blackpool Tower to the Eiffel Tower.

Someone (not sure who) once said, "Management is doing things right, leadership is doing the right things." "Efficiency is concerned with doing things right. Effectiveness is doing the right things." The latter is, I believe, attributed to Peter Drucker (management consultant, educator and author).

Retail was (as is now) a rapidly changing competitive environment (Retail is Detail) and it used to be a labour-intensive business requiring substantial numbers of staff to get the product to shelf

Pre-1980s stock replenishment consisted of large stockrooms in order to store several weeks' stock.

It, initially, involved manual counting of stock on a cyclic basis using stock books (which were lists of products stocked for each product category). I can still remember (sad I know) the formula applied for calculating an order as follows:

- $S(a) + O + O - 2S(b) = O(q)$
- S(a) was the physical stock count at the last count (say four weeks ago)
- O + O the last previous two order quantities added together
- − 2S(b) was taking away double of the latest stock count
- O(q) was the latest quantity of stock to be ordered

The order was then telephoned through to a direct supplier or written on stock cards and sent to Boots central warehouses for delivery. (This, as in other industries, was later to be replaced by computerised "just in time" replenishment.)

Also, Pre-1980s where this stock was displayed on a shelf, stock within a specific product category was essentially determined by the store manager based on sales volume and other principles such as "Eye level is Buy level" and if a product was available in different sizes then display the largest to the right. (As we read from left to right and so are more likely to purchase the larger product.)

During my time at Tamworth many systems changed to further centralisation. Ordering and stock counting was completed using pre-typed (computer generated) inventory lists which had a tear-off counterfoil attached, on which to enter the manual count. These counterfoils were then detached and sent via the internal post system for scanning by the Head Office computers. These were called ASCOT sheets (Automatic Stock Control and Ordering Techniques).

Another such set of sheets for seasonal stock were known as EPSOM sheets (Electronic Products Seasonal Ordering Method). You can just imagine the Head Office brainstorming sessions to come up with these titles (I guess all workplaces have such jargon).

Merchandising exact shelf position location of products were sent to be adhered to. These were called TRENT plans. Were these named after Lord Trent of Boots fame or the fact that Nottingham (Head Office) stands on the river TRENT? No of course not, it was "Total Remerchandising Employing New Techniques"!

Most central warehousing was located in Beeston, Nottingham, or Airdrie, Scotland, and bulk stock orders sent overnight via huge articulated lorries, to local distribution centres to be changed into smaller delivery vans which could navigate around the various UK High Streets. This stock movement still required large stockroom space in stores.

During my time at Tamworth, Boots trialled (piloted) the use of CSRs (Common Stock Rooms). This was a local warehouse which provided several nearby branches with daily stock deliveries from stock data entered into a "brick-like" hand terminal at each store transmitted via local networks to the warehouse. The aim was reduction in labour, stock investment and branch storage. A System which took many years to perfect as technology advanced. Perhaps Tamworth was chosen due to the area's logistics history.

You can see why my pharmacy role was diminished during this time. I did, however (despite me being non-political, or so I thought), become a local representative of the Boots Pharmacists' Association. BPA was formed in 1973 by Boots pharmacists for Boots pharmacists and is a listed trade union (its role is to offer advice on professional issues as well as representation in disciplinary and grievance meetings and legal protection). At the time that I was a rep (for four years) meetings could only be held on Sundays (then non-working days).

This non-political status was also put to the test as I was elected as an unpaid volunteer councillor to Austrey Parish Council (my arm was twisted by my neighbour, the Parish Clerk, over a pint in the Bird in Hand). The role meant commenting on planning applications, street cleaning, highways, street lighting and managing the budget (deciding how much to raise through council tax, known as the precept, to deliver the services needed in Austrey).

Socially, we both joined Tamworth Volleyball Club and actively played in the West Midlands Volleyball League.

During our summer camping trip to the Isle of Wight we tried our hands at windsurfing at Shanklin and I became hooked. (I continued avidly with this as well as the volleyball until I was unable, due to health, until April 2007.)

So we bought all the gear (boards, sails, wetsuits and buoyancy jackets etc.) and embarked on a RYA (Royal Yachting Association) course. The location of this course is quite unique (and may possibly come as a surprise to anyone reading this). It was on a lake reservoir in the middle of Spaghetti Junction, Aston Reservoir (also known as Salford Lake)! This reservoir was formerly used for drinking water from the river Tame and later as a boating lake though the latter is no longer the case.

We then proudly had our certificates and then joined Tamworth Windsurfing Club which was based at Borrowpit lake in the heart of Tamworth. The lake was originally dug to extract the aggregate when part of the ring road called "the egg" was being constructed.

I windsurfed on this lake in all weathers (hail rain and snow), even breaking ice in pursuit of this leisure activity. There were no changing facilities and so changing in and out of wetsuits could be "brass monkeys" at times. Even Elkie joined us many times on the board and many times swimming as Labradors do. The lake is nowadays exclusively for fishing.

As a club we also had many trips away, camping and sailing, and one such trip was to Bala Lake (Llyn Tegid Wales) where I nearly came a cropper. Bala lake is a freshwater glacial lake (whose source is the river Dee, which flows both in and out), over four miles long and a mile wide with a depth of 138ft. The water temperature is a cool average of 10C (ranging from 5C in February up to 15C late August). I can agree that it is cold and virtually pitch black one foot or more below the surface. On our first visit we stayed at the Glanllyn Caravan and camping park and launched from its private beach on the South West end of the lake.

I was a novice windsurfer and my maximum wind speed level was about Force 4 (a moderate breeze on the Beaufort scale). On this particular day as the wind was blowing a "huey" we all went out onto the water together (safety in numbers) but as the wind speed suddenly increased to Force7/8 (near gale/gale) I got blown downwind, separated from the group.

I beached, started the board and soon got motoring but as the wind gusted I dropped the sail. Then I was in trouble. As I kept standing up on the board trying to pull my mast and sail out of the water (uphaul) the waves would knock me off the board (as I was using my full body weight and arm strength and on the edge of the board). Sometimes I would catapult over the sail into the water and other times fall backwards into the water and get stuck under the sail underwater. This happened dozens of times and I began to get exhausted and probably hypothermic in the freezing cold, dark water.

Then the mast and sail separated from the board and panic started to set in and I had a choice: "Do I stay with the mast and sail or the board?" The RYA training kicked in and I initially stayed with the board floating in the water trying to get some breath and energy, yet I was getting colder and colder and shivering so I decided to swim 25 yards or so to collect my mast and sail which were hanging in the water like a huge anchor. The next job was to swim back to the board (with sail in tow) which had inadvertently drifted further away and then release the sail from the mast boom (by releasing the outhaul rope from its cleat). Once this was achieved the sail had to be rolled up and the boom released from the mast and then all the components secured on top of the board. This again was exhausting and many times I had to hold onto the board to stop myself slipping away into that dark and cold water (and I thought I would drown).

Climbing on top of the board was an onerous task which I managed to complete on several occasions only to be dumped unceremoniously back in the drink. This seemed to take hours. The times I managed to stay on the board resting it was difficult to appreciate the breathtaking, tranquil mountain backdrop and the "chuffing" steam trains of the Bala Lake Railway. At this point I had floated opposite Llangower point, which at the time had a catamaran club I could just see in the distance (at least half a mile away). On the beach area of the club I could just make out a couple sitting on deckchairs with binoculars.

*

This reminded me of the hilarious Public Information Film (1970s) *Joe and Petunia – Coastguard* in which they were watching a dinghy sailor in trouble and saying things like "he's taking a swim now", "he must know us he's shouting at us" and "he's waving at us now, Petunia" (worth a view on YouTube).

Back to the seriousness of my situation, I clambered

onto the board and shouted and crossed my arms on my chest and into the air, recognised as the international distress standard (as learnt on our RYA course). Nothing happened and no one came to rescue me so I had a further choice to make: "Do I swim dragging board and gear across the half mile to the catamaran club or do I try and stay on the board and hopefully drift downwind the three miles to the North end of the lake near Bala Town and civilisation?" As I said, panic was setting in together with hypothermia and as I could see shore, I decided on the swim.

I eventually made it to the shore (grateful of the many swimming miles put in as a youngster at Bishop Auckland Swimming Club and at Longfield Comprehensive School, making me a reasonably strong swimmer). On the shore I just collapsed on my back and heard the couple say, "We thought you were struggling!"

Carol had been panicking back at the campsite and asking other windsurfers if they had seen me as they said they had lost sight of me. She (pregnant and with two dogs in the car boot) then frantically drove 14 miles around the lake searching for me. Now the problem is that at many parts around the lake you cannot actually see the lake from the road. Even when you could it was hard to see a windsurfer in the dark choppy waters from such a distance (despite my black with fluorescent pink and green striped wet suit). Thankfully, Carol eventually found me "laid out"(though alive) on the Catamaran Club Beach.

The whole experience taught me to respect how the weather can suddenly change tranquil waters such as sea, lakes and rivers into dangerous cauldrons of freezing cold water.

Many years later this came home to roost, tragically involving one of my son Lewis's friends. Lewis has grown up to be an extremely proficient windsurfer and sailed in many famous windsurfing locations in France, Spain and Italy etc. and ventures out in only high winds with short sails and short wide low volume boards which need a strong wind to keep the surfer up on the water surface.

Proficient windsurfers are excellent waterstarters (an essential technique which allows you to be pulled up onto the board from a lying in the water position), something I never mastered.

Lewis had gone, with eight or so experienced windsurfers, on a very windy winter's day to surf from Cockerham Sands near the Lune Estuary, Morecambe Bay (this being very tidal you can only sail two hours either side of high tide). Then suddenly when they were on the water the wind dropped and the fog rolled in leaving them stranded in the water. All but one somehow managed to get to shore, they all attempted to rescue him but were thwarted by the lack of visibility. Their friend shouted to them, "Save yourselves I will get back" (he was the most experienced windsurfer of them all, many years under his belt and a very experienced boat sailor too, who knew the waters the best) but sadly he couldn't. So they called the coastguard and rescue services and stood vigil for many hours calling out and waiting for the rescuers. A large scale air and sea search, in terrible conditions, was conducted even through the night but tragically he was found washed up on Middleton Sands in Morecambe Bay the following day. He had, so tragically, been swept to his death by a powerful ebb tide. **RIP**.

Lewis, Carol and I along with his windsurfing fraternity attended his funeral. A stark reminder if ever needed to take care. Lewis now windsurfs with a GPS alarm responder which sends an international emergency distress signal to the coastguard.

Time to return back to the more pleasant time in Austrey. Further back in my story I referred to both "a doggy tale" and "two dogs in the boot" but I have only so far told you about Elkie. We had long working days when Elkie was in the house alone, of course with plenty of space food and water but nonetheless lonely.

So one day at Christmas time I dropped Carol off at Tamworth station saying that I needed the car to collect a Christmas tree. However, once she was entrenched into the train I drove off to the nearest dog rescue centre looking for company for Elkie. There were many differing breeds and sizes and I had no preconception what type I was looking for when this medium-sized dog came running up to me brushing my legs, wagging its tail and looking at me with sad pleading eyes. I immediately and soft heartedly thought this is the one and so she was bundled into the hatch boot of the car and off we went for the Christmas tree.

It then came time to pick Carol up from the station. As she was getting into the car I said, "Have a look in the boot, what do you think about the Christmas tree?" Then out popped the head of this bedraggled dog with the pleading eyes.

The dog was a black, tan and white cross between a wire-haired terrier and a Jack Russell terrier (a right Heinz '57 mix). Her hair was so spiky that we named her "Toyah" (after Toyah Wilcox the punk-funky style singer), a great pal for Elkie.

In fact they were friends instantly and became partners in crime many a time and Toyah was extremely loyal and protective (I think she knew she had been rescued). We had a public footpath at the side of our house with a high corresponding brick wall bordering our garden which the dogs couldn't get over. However, they could jump on top of the coal bunker barking and peering over giving many a walker a shock.

Whilst in Austrey I took up cricket again (I used to play for many years as a child and played for my school team and in fact had a couple of games playing for Darlington as a schoolboy). This revelation came about again in the "Bird in Hand" after a few sessions of Marston's Pedigree. The village did not have a cricket team so a bunch of us decided to set up one. We named it Austrey Amblers Cricket Club in recognition of the fact that we did not have a ground and played all our games away or used the nearby Newton Regis cricket club ground when they didn't have a home match. On latter occasions Carol and the other lads' wives made excellent home-made teas.

This resulted in being on another committee (as Treasurer) along with my roles on the Tamworth Volleyball Club Committee (player coach, sometimes as chairman and sometimes as treasurer) and also a role on the Tamworth Windsurfing Club. How on earth did I find time for work?

It was a lot easier in that Carol participated both in windsurfing and volleyball and with no kids yet on the horizon. At work I was getting itchy feet and even contemplated leaving Boots and joining in a partnership with another pharmacist to joint own a couple of pharmacies in Derby.

However, I found myself on the "promotion list" again and this time (November 1985) was appointed as Store Manager of Boots Wylde Green (The Lanes shopping centre, Sutton Coldfield). This was to be my first solo management role and as it was a smaller store I returned to an increased pharmacist role too.

This store was much closer to Carol's place of work resulting in significantly less commuting into the centre of Birmingham. It meant another move of house, but not too far this time and it enabled us to keep playing volleyball for Tamworth, and windsurfing as well as cricket for me. We were to become 021ees named after the telephone STD for Birmingham (now 0121). So it was that we put our Austrey home on the market.

As I needed to be local to my place of work (for alarm call out purposes), we managed to find a new home in Wylde Green itself, a lovely leafy suburb of Sutton Coldfield which in the 16th century was an area of common barren land known as "the Wyld" and sparsely populated. However, when we moved there it was a "middle class working area with housing stock dating from the late 1930s to late 1940s" and, in 1974, had become part of the city of Birmingham along with the rest of Sutton Coldfield. Wylde Green and its neighbour Boldmere had a convenient set of amenities of shops, pubs, obligatory curry houses and train stations on our doorstep.

The area was (and still is) served by the Redditch-Birmingham New Street-Lichfield Cross-City line for rapid and easy commuting into Birmingham city centre (very convenient for Carol too). Wylde Green was also on the Erdington/Aston border of Birmingham, bounded by the Chester road.

Elkie and Toyah (our dogs) were also well catered for due to the fact that we were in easy walking distance of Sutton Park (consisting of 465 acres of lowland heathland comprising of wet and dry heathland areas, bog, mire, acid grassland, and seven lakes). Many features of Sutton Park date back over thousands of years, including the Neolithic (6000 years ago), Bronze (3000 years ago), and Iron Ages. Sutton Park's Roman road known as "Ryknield Street" is 1.5 miles long, built as part of the Roman conquest of the West Midlands, just after the Roman army landed in Kent in AD 43. Some of the lakes were man made (by damming small streams) in the Middle Ages to help feed the local population. Bream, baked in flour and seasoned with spice, pepper, saffron, cloves and cinnamon, was a favourite at the time.

By 1985 Carol had moved from NACRO Highgate South Birmingham and became Development Officer for NACRO Aston North Birmingham. 1985 was another year of racial tension which led to the second Handsworth riots (the first being 1981) and caused tensions and difficulties at her workplace and local area, within the black and Asian communities therein. The riots accounted for two deaths (two brothers burnt to death in the post office that they ran), two other people unaccounted for, 35 injured, 45 shops looted and burnt, and a trail of damage running into thousands of pounds. Consequently, more than 1500 police officers were drafted into the area. As well as racial tension, unemployment was seen as a major factor (Handsworth having had one of the highest unemployment rates in Birmingham, and fewer than 5% of black pupils to have left school in the summer preceding the riot had found employment.

On a lighter note I took up squash again (having played regularly as a teenager and almost daily whilst at Bradford University) as another sport and we became members of North Birmingham Squash Club trying to remain fit and healthy (in fact during our time in Ipswich and Austrey I had not needed to avail the NHS of its GP services) although that was to change.

I had been having recurrent fevers and sore throats and noticed swellings on both sides of the tongue and so visited the GP. He looked into my throat and saw the swellings and became concerned as to what was causing it since my tonsils had been removed when I was a child. Because of this I was then referred to an ENT consultant for further investigation, as he was concerned it may be cancerous. Of course this set off alarm and distress for us. However, the consultant put our minds at ease as he said that he thought the swellings were infected sublingual tonsils but if they didn't recede after another course of antibiotics then surgery and a biopsy would be necessary. Apparently the "tonsils" we all know are in fact palatine tonsils and are located on the sides of the throat and seen when we open our mouths. We all do, however, also have tonsils located on the back of the tongue as well which are almost never removed in childhood tonsillectomies. Lingual tonsillitis is a rare cause of sore throat and two thirds of patients are reported to have a history of palatine tonsillectomy or adenoidectomy and other potential causes include lymphoma and chronic infection.

These back of the tongue swellings did not recede, so pre-Christmas week 1987 I was admitted, with an overnight stay, to East Birmingham Hospital and had them removed by cryotherapy knife (freezing to destroy the diseased tissue) together with a biopsy sample. We then had a couple of anxious weeks to await results. The post-operative recovery meant that (at the busiest time of the year for my store) I needed two weeks' sick leave.

Fortunately the results were negative and therefore no cancerous tissue found, but what a worry! (Though nothing in comparison to what would befall us in later years.)

It was time to settle down!

Carol and I decided to have a family, and (like many couples I'm sure) it didn't go straight to plan which led to a degree of anxiety and concern. We tried using fertility thermometers and corresponding graph charts plotting to check for ovulation. Science was also moving forward in that home ovulation testing kits became available to purchase from pharmacies, and even with my Boots Staff discount this was proving to be costly and certainly an unromantic by-the-clock experience! Our GP then referred us to the Fertility Clinic and we then both had to have our fertilities checked, another experience! Our hearts go out to anyone with fertility issues. Anyway we attended the local hospital to see the specialist consultant, armed with graphs and charts. The consultant gave us the good news that our fertility checks were ok and he then tore up all the sheets and said "just go home relax and let it happen".

So it was that Carol became pregnant, expecting our first child, due September 1988, and she enjoyed watching the Seoul 1988 Summer Olympics whilst on maternity leave. I of course kept "soldiering on" being a pharmacist and Store Manager together with the long hours and varied work that entailed.

I had always wanted a top of the range professional type table football table and my good friend, who was in the gaming industry, managed to secure one for me at a reduced cost. However this was soon blocked with the simple words: "We can't afford it. We need to buy a pram and cot." Dash it!

Carol developed a craving for American Style Cream Soda pop which at all hours I could be found roaming the local stores for a bottle (or two) of. I also prepared myself by reading midwifery handbooks and manuals (supplied by, my midwife sister-in-law) which in hindsight was disturbing overkill.

Then one night in September her "waters" broke in the wee small hours. Panic of course then set in. I had the store keys and the "golden key" and had to pass them on!

Consequently before driving Carol to Birmingham Queen Elizabeth Hospital, at break neck speed (as a first timer I thought I didn't have much time to spare), I had to drop the keys off "en route".

Why the rush? Poor Carol was in labour for 36 hours and it wasn't until later the following evening that our first child was born.

During the birth, in a very hot and sunny maternity ward, I was stood at "the business end" when the midwife shouted, "We need to do an urgent episiotomy and we don't have time for local anaesthetic." To my horror they then took the scissors and cut the perineum and blood flowed followed by our son "poppng out". Crikey, she was so brave.

So our son Lewis came into the world born a "Brummie".

I did, like many new fathers, have the opportunity to cut the umbilical cord (so all my University dissection techniques were not fully wasted).

Still I managed to work, windsurf, play cricket and squash (how I don't know looking back) and we had to change our hatch back car for an estate to accommodate Lewis and the two dogs.

I was also getting "itchy feet" again and toyed with the idea of buying a pharmacy in Shanklin (Isle of Wight) and decided against it as the goodwill alone was £250,000 and interest rates at around 14% (in those days a new pharmacy could not be opened within two miles of existing pharmacies and so existing shops with NHS pharmacy contracts demanded a high premium with much profit to be made by selling to the "Big Boy" multiples). It would have also meant living in a tiny flat above the shop. Altogether not practicable with a new baby and two dogs! Good for windsurfing though!

However, I was then back on the promotion list. So much so in fact that I had successful interviews for three stores within a week, those being Wantage (Oxfordshire), Whitby (North Yorkshire) and Retford (Nottinghamshire). What a decision to make for our family. When I went for the Wantage interview we took Lewis along for the weekend, stopping in a local B&B above a pub and went reviewing house prices. Another shock! The housing stock was greatly inflated compared to "Brum". Not only that, but Carol also went around the local retail shops to do a shopping survey of a weekly basket of goods. This, along with the price of a pint of beer, showed us that (much like today's prices) we could not afford to live in beautiful Oxfordshire without much sacrifice.

Whitby is such a lovely place to live, being a nostalgic seaside location (Dracula fame) in the beautiful North Yorkshire moors. It was the smallest store of the three and I was keen to progress within Boots (and perhaps we would have been reluctant to move on from there) so we chose the largest store Retford.

So once again it was time to sell the house, "up sticks" and commute, this time leaving Carol at home, not just one dog this time but two, as well as our three month old baby son, Lewis!

So it was back to travelling on Monday and Thursday mornings and Saturday evening and stopping in a hotel on Monday, Tuesday, Thursday and Friday nights.

Sometimes I travelled to Retford on a Sunday night, having put Lewis to bed following a bedtime story. One particular night April 8th January was memorable for the wrong reason, this being the Kegworth air disaster. A Boeing 737-400 crashed onto the motorway embankment between the M1 motorway and the A453 road near Kegworth at 20:24 hours with 47 deaths, 74 injuries and thankfully 79 survivors (including the eight crew). How it had managed to just miss the actual motorway is perhaps a miracle.

I had just passed this very point on the motorway five minutes previously! Best not to dwell on this and just to be so thankful.

Back to Retford (also known as East Retford), again a historical market town and indeed one of the oldest English market towns having been granted its first charter in 1105. Interestingly, Retford is known as being at the centre of nonconformism, with the origins of Pilgrims, Baptists and Wesleyans being in this area. Not sure the latter three apply to me but a nonconformist maybe.

Artefacts from the Mesolithic and Neolithic (New Stone Age) periods have been found in the area together with evidence of Viking and Roman settlements. Modern history shows that Retford was bombed six times in World War Two and though it was on the bombing route to high value targets such as Sheffield, it was also protected by many surrounding air force bases.

I think I was appointed to the Retford store (in Carolgate, East Retford) by serendipity as the previous manager was also called John Atkinson, so they didn't even need to change the name on the manager's office door! I'm sure it confused several of the regular customers when they came in asking to speak to the pharmacist "John Atkinson" and out from the dispensary I popped. It was a busy store especially on open-air market days. I was also a tutor/mentor for my third pre-registration graduate (the other two being at Wylde Green), helping her develop skills learnt at University and hopefully passing on some knowledge and wisdom. In fact she was a star graduate and it was a pleasure to recommend her entry onto the Royal Pharmaceutical Society Register.

So in April 1989 we moved into our new home in the outskirts of Retford. The timing is memorable, unfortunately, as it was around the time of the Hillsborough disaster (15th April 1989) at which there was a fatal human crush during the football match between Liverpool and Nottingham Forest at Hillsborough Stadium in nearby Sheffield. This has been well documented over succeeding years, with several public enquiries as there were 97 deaths and 766 injuries caused by overcrowding of supporters into enclosed pens within the ground.

Socially I joined Retford Volleyball Club, playing in the East Midlands League, and a local windsurfing club at a nearby private lake, as well as the local snooker club (which was very well utilised when my father-in-law visited). Carol became a full-time mum at home for Lewis and then Sean (more of that soon) visiting many mother, baby and toddler groups and enjoying many a coffee morning at friends' houses.

December 1989 was a very cold winter in the East Midlands and in one week particularly, the temperatures plummeted to −20C, and an Artic storm rolled in causing atmospheric icing. This caused super cooling of water droplets and heavy and sudden ice build-up on the main electricity power lines and pylons around Retford. The massive sudden ice load caused catastrophic failure of the overhead lines. Five out of six pylons, which supplied all the electricity to the area's National Grid, collapsed and folded like a pack of cards leaving Retford and the immediate area without any electricity for five days! This caused challenges at work and home alike. We had gas central heating at home but of course run by electric pumps and thermostats and at minus 20 the house was bitterly cold. Not only that, but our cooker was electric! We did, however, have a gas fire in the lounge and so that's where we all slept, on the floor, at night in the lounge. Fifteen-month-old baby Lewis, Carol (now pregnant again with number two), myself and two dogs. For hot water and food we boiled pans on a two ring gas camping stove. It was a real "blitz" style mentality with lighting by torch and candlelight. After five days the novelty had completely worn off.

The difficulty with work was figuring out how to operate an essential dispensing pharmacy service for the public without electric and lights.

We had a small portable petrol generator which ran a small string of about six light bulbs under which we could just about read the prescriptions and see stock and were therefore able to run an effective but limited service for patients. However, the cash tills were all electric and the cash drawers could only be opened using a manual crank handle. When a customer brought goods to checkout we had to list everything on paper and add up the items manually using a calculator and hope the customers had near enough the correct change to pay. Credit cards could be used but the "old way" using imprinter rollers and carbonated paper slips. It wasn't altogether fool proof as the calculators were solar powered and needed sunlight and so we needed to quickly purchase battery operated ones.

Another problem was how to obtain petrol for our portable generator as all the petrol stations within an 18 mile radius were down as the pumps needed electricity with which to dispense fuel. Fortunately my boss (District Manager) lived in Lincoln and was able to obtain a full petrol can for our "gennie" and car. All of my staff were brilliant coping in such challenging circumstances and coming to work and providing a service for the public.

Late March 1990 the volleyball league season was in its final week and we were placed second in the league behind Derby Fire Service with one more match to play, it was against Derby themselves and the winners would be league champions. As player coach I had a big responsibility, so Carol (heavily pregnant), baby Lewis and I travelled separately from the other five members of the team, we could only just muster a team of six (the minimum required).

The game itself was tense, and exciting, and we were winning two sets to one and going into the final set. We were then winning this set by three points when I went up for a block at the net (middle position) and as I landed I heard a loud "crack" as I landed; I had broken my ankle. There was a technical timeout called to check my injury, but as I was rolling in pain and couldn't stand, the sports centre staff called an ambulance. The ambulance crew then offered us a choice of Derby hospital or Nottingham QE hospital, we chose the latter as it was probably easier to get home from there. Carol had to then try and fit in behind the driver's wheel (together with her large bump), bundle Lewis into the car and follow the ambulance to the hospital (in the days before satellite navigation). If this wasn't bad enough we lost the game by default (as the rules stated because we didn't have any substitutes) and of course lost the league!

At the hospital the X-ray confirmed a broken ankle and it was placed in a plaster cast and crutches issued. This was going to be an inconvenience for Carol, home and work. As far as work was concerned I contacted Head Office and managed to arrange collection of a demonstration wheelchair from the Beeston, Nottingham warehouse (as we sold them as a company) to use for work. I was then able to go to work in the wheelchair and manage the store whilst locum pharmacists "ran" the dispensary. For health and safety liability this had to be undertaken at my own risk, such was my dedication to the cause. My staff were very good at arranging a rota to pick me up from and drop me back at home on a daily basis in order that Carol (heavily pregnant) and with a toddler was not "dragged" out of the house to get me to work.

Then one Tuesday my dad visited from the North East to mow our lawns as Carol couldn't manage the mower and I, of course, had the "pot" on my foot.

There was quite a decent-sized lawn at the rear, large enough for an outdoor volleyball court and net (which we played on many a family occasion) which needed attention. Having completed this my dad then went with Carol, and Lewis in his pushchair, to walk our dogs Elkie and Toyah down the country lane beside our road. It was on this early evening walk that Carol's waters broke (upon return to the house this was confirmed by a test kit, supplied by Sue, Carol's midwife sister)!

I am not so sure out of the three of us who was panicking the most as to what to do next, as this was happening three weeks early. So Sue and my mother-in-law were telephoned. They set off from the North East and my dad drove Carol and I, together with Lewis, to Worksop maternity hospital. Carol was duly examined, as well as being admitted. We were then told that as nothing was going to happen imminently we should go home. So my dad drove me and Lewis home, by which time Sue and her mam had arrived. Then at 5am Wednesday morning (Carol had to convince the midwives that the birth was now imminent) I received a telephone call requesting me to return to the hospital. My dad then drove me back with crutches and wheelchair in tow.

We arrived just before 6am and our new son Sean was born at 6.19am, Wednesday 11th April and, on my birthday! (We had made it just in time.) We already had the name "Joseph" chosen but as the midwife asked, "What are you calling him?" I replied, "Sean." So he was now Sean Joseph. (Lewis and Sean are both derivatives of John.) When Sean was going to be 18 years old I would be 50 on the same day!

We visited again the next day early evening for visiting and I just happened to sit beside Carol and the bed with my broken ankle, in its pot up on the bed. A nurse approached and by the look in her eye I thought I was going to get a right telling off. However, to our surprise, the words that she spoke were, "You poor thing, would you like a cup of tea?"

So we now had two children and two dogs, and in October1990 I was asked to attend a three week "leadership" residential course, including two of three weekends based at the Kegworth Hotel and Conference Centre. Poor Carol again left at home with the two dogs and a toddler and a baby.

The course included several psychological assessments, presentation skills, advertising, sales promotion and merchandising skills, also business strategic thinking, strategy formulation, planning and evaluation. Other elements included specialist selling skills training, incorporating local demographic and competitor analysis. This course was facilitated by external consultants and was not just about being fed information, you had to go and find out about it through research and interviews. Interviews were arranged by ourselves but from a list of key Company Directors, Business Unit Managers, Area Managers, Head Office Trainers etc. The interviews were conducted in teams of three (each having to complete at least six interviews and the results fed back to the rest of the group). Just like an early version of "the Apprentice" I guess. On one of our interviews my colleague got the interview time completely mixed up and didn't realise until we were travelling across Nottingham that we should have started the interview in two minutes' time! Impossible to achieve so we decided upon the ruse to say that we had a puncture and would be late. It of course backfired on us as the

Operations Director didn't like to be kept waiting and so kept us waiting 90 minutes outside his office. We thought our careers would be curtailed! Not only that but at the start of each answer to our questions he would use a quotation from an encyclopaedic book of quotations on his desk.

It was all very intensive and heavy going but we did have some team building exercises built into the programme. One such occasion was to visit the Nottingham Goose Fair.

The name "Goose Fair" comes from the fact that thousands of geese were driven from the Lincolnshire fens to be sold in Nottingham.

In 1284 a Royal charter was granted for city fairs in Nottingham, mainly started as a livestock and trade event, with a reputation for its excellent cheese but today it is now known for its fairground attractions and rides that attract many thousands of visitors each year. We let our "hair down" on many a ride.

The completion of this course then led from 7th January 1991 (Carol's birthday) to my next 38 week temporary appointment as District Manager covering Lincolnshire and South Yorkshire and as such diversifying slightly away from pure pharmacy (although I was responsible, in a senior management role, for all pharmacists, managers and staff within the district). The stores I had to visit and oversee on a regular two weekly basis (dependent upon need and circumstance) included Doncaster, Thorne, Scunthorpe, Brigg Grimsby and Cleethorpes in the North. Then Retford, Gainsborough, Market Rasen, Louth and Skegness in the middle. And then Newark on Trent, and Sleaford in the South, quite some area. This role certainly "opened my eyes" as you like to think that stores within the same company work to the same standard but this was definitely not the case.

Any serious customer complaints or dispensing errors by any of the staff had to be investigated by me and appropriate action taken and in some cases leading to disciplinary procedures and dismissal (which was not easy with my former colleague store managers, but that was my role).

There were no mobile phones but we did have "pagers" which beeped an electronic message and phone number to call from the nearest telephone call box or store depending upon the urgency of the message. My line manager used to "bleep" me frequently at around 5pm on a Friday to ensure that I was still working. He would also regularly attend with me when he was out on store visits with Head Office personnel which you could guarantee would always be a Friday as he loved "Fish and Chip Friday" and we had some of the best fish shops on his patch (Cleethorpes, Grimsby and Louth).

During May 1991 we had worrying times with both Lewis and Sean having illnesses which made us reassess perspectives. Firstly Lewis developed a chest infection and acute asthma attack which led to serious breathing difficulties and hospitalisation. He was admitted to hospital for a week for nebulisation and oxygen ventilation. This resulted with me stopping (sleeping) overnight by his hospital bedside and then Carol taking over during the day whilst I went to work. Fortunately after a week he fully recovered and returned home. As all parents know child illness causes anxiety.

Chapter 8

North East Return

I was at the bottom of the garden, shortly after Lewis came home, when I heard Carol scream and bang on the bathroom window. Sean was being bathed when suddenly he stopped breathing and started to turn blue. Carol managed to get him breathing again and we took him urgently to see the GP who in no uncertain terms told us to take him straight to hospital pronto. Sean was then examined, given oxygen, steroids and nebulisation and also kept in hospital for a week so we repeated the day/night routine.

Fortunately Sean also fully recovered. Lewis had developed asthma (triggered by infections) as did Sean (triggered by over exertion and excessive exercise). They were, many years later, fortunate to both "grow" out of it.

So, during my final few weeks of my successful District Manager role I was again on the promotion list and consequently on the move again! This time was different in that we wanted to return as close as possible to our families (in the North East) for support. I applied for a parallel move to Bishop Auckland, County Durham and was successful. The Area Manager who interviewed me questioned me at the time as to why I was applying for a store that was not seen as a promotion for me and so I explained my personal reasons that it was solely for the benefit of my family. The Area Manager's interview report stated, "His previous experience in a similar store and his energetic approach make him an ideal candidate for this store with its inherent problems." These problems were just the retail economic problems of the time and a staff morale issue. So on October 1ˢᵗ 1991 I started in Bishop Auckland and "hit the road" again, leaving Carol once again home alone with the lads and dogs five days a week and three nights as I trundled up the A1 to the North East. This time, I had no need to stop in a swanky and lonely hotel as I could stay with my parents in nearby Darlington.

Bishop Auckland (originally known as "Alclit" or rock above the river but also Aukland in Norse meaning additional land referring to extra land given to the Bishop of Durham by King Canute around 1020AD) was also linked with the close by settlements of St Helen Auckland, West Auckland and St Andrew Auckland (an old name for South Church) all of which are along the path of the river Gaunless. The origin of the river name is old Norse meaning useless (due to its inability to power a mill, sustain fish or create fertile floodplains). Its early history links with the Bishops of Durham and the establishment of Auckland Castle as the main residence of Durham's Bishops. Auckland Castle was also a look-out post for the Romans at nearby Binchester (of our engagement fame). The industrial revolution, as coal mining took hold, led to a rapidly growing town culminating at the start of the twentieth century with 16,000 people in the local area being employed in the mining industry. Traditionally "Bishop" had a strong retail presence and became one of Durham County's main population centres with good bus and rail connections and thriving markets on Thursdays and Saturdays (to which many shoppers from surrounding smaller settlements, on the Durham coalfield, flocked). However, the last deep colliery in the area closed in 1968 and this, along with increased car ownership and competition from local shopping malls such as the Metro Centre in Gateshead together with Teeside Park, led to a rapid decline in "Bishop's" retail environment. It was against this backdrop that it was my challenge to improve store sales!

High unemployment together with increased deprivation also led to increased criminality and we "struggled" with a high degree of shoplifting for which we had to be forever vigilant. One of my first tasks involved changing the layout of the store to improve customer "traffic" flow and to introduce new ranges. Refitting the store meant disposal of old fittings, we didn't need to invest in many skips because as soon as we filled them the "locals" just came and helped themselves negating any requirement to empty them.

Just another anecdote on this criminality links both the local area (West Auckland) and pharmacy history to the notorious murderer Mary Ann Cotton aka "The Dark Angel" the County Durham serial killer. It is thought that she may have had as many as 21 victims including three of her four husbands and 11 of her 13 children. She used arsenic to poison her victims, administered in a comforting cup of tea made in a small teapot (now in Beamish Museum) reserved for the purpose. She was convicted and hanged in 1873 for the murder of her stepson. Whilst she manly lived and conducted herself in Northumberland she rekindled a romance with her former lover Joseph Nattrass (who lived in West Auckland) and persuaded her family to move there. Her demise came at the hands of West Auckland's assistant coroner and parish official Thomas Riley who asked her to help nurse a child sick with smallpox. She complained that her stepson "was in the way" and asked Riley if he could be committed to the workhouse but Riley told her she would have to accompany her stepson to said workhouse. She then told that him that he was a sickly boy and said, "I won't be troubled long. He'll go like all the rest of the

Cottons." Five days later the boy died and Riley informed the police. Investigations took place and local newspapers took up the story and discovered that Mary Ann had moved around North East England and had "lost" three husbands, a lover, a friend, mother and 11 children all of whom had died of "stomach fevers".

In 1851 The Arsenic Act was passed (at the time arsenic was widely used as a pigment and in agricultural products such as sheep dressings). The Act was introduced to regulate its sale (requiring sellers to maintain a written and signed record to whom they had sold arsenic and it had to be coloured with either soot or indigo) as well as addressing increasing public concern over accidental and deliberate arsenic poisonings. This was replaced by the Pharmacy and Poisons Act 1933 (mentioned earlier in my story).

It was early November 1991 that we moved into our new house on the outer boundary of Bishop Auckland and West Auckland near the village of Escomb (which has a church built in the seventh century that has been called "England's earliest complete church"). Later on Lewis was attending his first school at Escomb Primary School and Sean attended Aclet (that Norse derivative again) Nursery School, Bishop Auckland, along with his cousin and partner in crime, Mathew (my brother Steve and his wife Sue, and their two sons Mathew and David lived in Bishop Auckland too).

Late April 1992 we were both delighted to discover that Carol was pregnant again and that we were expecting our third child and we seemed to be settling down. Sean and Lewis's asthma was improving and being controlled, yet we still had a few scares particularly with Lewis. After a few late night call-outs (as a result of their acute asthma attacks) our GP recommended that we obtain a home nebuliser and gave us a letter to enable it to happen.

As a pharmacist I was able to purchase one from the manufacturer (via our drug wholesaler). The GP also prescribed an emergency supply of oral dissolvable steroids and nebuliser bronchodilator solutions. These were to be kept in the house to be used in an emergency as necessary (our GP knowing that with our past experiences and my job as a pharmacist that we would only use them appropriately and only when necessary). This enabled us to manage their attacks without need for hospitalisation.

Unfortunately on **May 14th** 1992 (the day and month forever embellished in our minds for reasons that will become self-evident later) Carol suffered a heavy bleed and subsequent miscarriage and was admitted to hospital. I drove her to hospital and was so unfocussed (full of feelings of extreme anxiety and palpitations and worry for Carol) that in the hospital car park I reversed into a post and put a large "V" dent in the boot of our new Ford Orion car (an insignificant event in the scheme of things).

Carol had to have an emergency surgical operation and this was also particularly distressing for her as the hospital staff did not explain what was happening and that did not become apparently clear until after the surgery.

The loss was devastating for us both and took us a period of time to recover from. We know that many people have unfortunately been through this trauma though it is of little comfort to be in that "club" when it happens to you. It is empathetic to talk about it though and our thoughts go out to those with such a dreadful experience. Fortunately all our family, friends and neighbours were a great support.

We then had to support each other and pragmatically get on with our lives. It was then back to work for me and back to caring and looking after the lads for Carol. We always had the boys' cousins, neighbours and friends' children around playing in "the close" as well as in our back garden (a regular kindergarten at which Carol thrived). Never a dull moment. Being so busy helped.

One of the roles undertaken throughout my pharmacy career has been the domiciliary supply of oxygen to patients, and even more so around Bishop Auckland. As previously mentioned the area had been a significant mining area and with that came associated health problems such as lung disorders.

The oxygen supply system worked by GPs prescribing and writing a prescription for an oxygen giving set (which is an attachment connector and regulatory valve with tubing and face mask) and up to a maximum of three oxygen cylinders (1360 Litre). The giving sets had to be purchased by the pharmacy and a monthly rental for each claimed back from the NHS, so only a finite number could be agreed to be stocked and afforded for each pharmacy. The cylinders were delivered direct from BOC (on account), full exchanged for empties on a one for one basis. The NHS then re-imbursed the pharmacy for the cost of actual gas supplied to each patient and an allowance (pence per mile) for delivery to the patient.

As a pharmacist I would visit and deliver (always after work) the sets, masks and oxygen as a first visit to a new patient, in order to set up the system, explain to the patient how to use, correctly and safely and how to swap empty for new cylinders and to check the oxygen flow rate setting (either two litres per minute or four). A 2Lpm setting would provide enough oxygen for around 11 hours. Subsequent replacement cylinders were delivered by store staff and sometimes via taxi.

We used to supply to patients' homes as well as nursing and residential homes. On one occasion I visited an elderly patient in Tow Law (up in the Wear valley) for a review, as they had been using exceptional amounts of oxygen. When I entered the patient's lounge there they were, surrounded by empty cylinders and one with an open valve, sitting whilst merrily puffing away on a cigarette. After switching off the valve and extolling the virtues of not smoking for the health of their lungs and for safety reasons, especially with bottled open oxygen cylinders around I "legged" it so we all didn't go up in flames together! The next day I contacted their GP so that their situation could be monitored.

Whilst at "Bishop" I became the company representative on the Durham Local Pharmaceutical Committee (more politics) until 1995 (4 years) and later for eight more years on the South Cumbria LPC. The role of the LPC (as an independent group representing community pharmacists and pharmacy owners) is to work locally with NHS England Area Teams, Care Commissioning groups, Local Authorities and other healthcare professionals to help plan healthcare services. It also negotiates and discusses pharmacy services with commissioners and liaises closely with their medical equivalents (the Local Medical Committee, Local Dental Committees and Local Optical Committees) to work together to deliver services to patients. This involved monthly or bi-monthly meetings or more if you were co-opted onto a working party. In essence it was the local arm of the national Pharmacy Services Negotiating Committee whose main function is to negotiate remuneration for services provided by pharmacies with the NHS. It might sound jargonistic and boring, but it was a part of my extended pharmacist role (and an essential and unseen bulwark to the NHS).

Socially, whilst we lived in "Bishop" we enjoyed many extended family (as they were all now local) occasions and many a party and social gathering with neighbours and friends. Our next door neighbour had converted his double garage to a bar and so several party nights were held there as well as the frequent sojourn to the local pub. I also became a member of the local pub quiz team.

I also joined the Haughton Volleyball Club (in Darlington) and played in the Tyneside and Teeside Volleyball League. This resulted in excellent friendships being formed that are still maintained to this day, together with many a social event, including camping (home and abroad) trips.

We bought our first caravan (progressing from tents to trailer tent to caravan) and stored it on a farm in Toronto (no not Canada as that a bit too far away, but only one mile away, incidentally named after the Canadian city after a coal baron with land in County Durham was visiting the said city when he learnt that coal had been discovered under his land. He therefore decided to call the mine Toronto, whence the village took its name).

We also regularly walked our dogs and took the boys (friends and cousins etc. at times) to Hamsterley Forest for an extensive workout (a great place for walking, horse riding and mountain biking). Hamsterley Forest (some 4,900 acres) was planted in the 1930s and tracks were built by unemployed men supplied through the Ministry of Labour, with most coming from the mining communities and shipyards of the North East. They were basically work camps where unemployed men carried out heavy labour. Some huts can still be seen today with the visitor centre being part of a prisoner of war camp during the Second World War.

It was on such a day out that we found on return to home that all the boys newly washed clothes had been stolen off the line (more criminality)! These were hard times for the North East.

On another occasion, the night before we were due to embark on our summer holiday with our caravan to the North Yorkshire moors, we were about to pack our car and we decided not to pack the car until the morning (before collecting the caravan from storage).

The following morning I looked out of the window and there was no car on the drive. I asked Carol whether she had put it in the garage and when she said she hadn't we realised it had been stolen. The boys were devastated that they couldn't go on their much anticipated holiday adventure. We contacted the local police and they put out a search for it. In the meantime Carol's dad (Tony) said that he would tow our caravan (he was also a caravanner) to our holiday destination the next day so that the boys could still have their holiday. What a star.

The police called the next morning and said to Carol those immortal lines, "Do you want the good news or the bad news?" Followed by, "The good news is that we have found your car but the bad news is that it doesn't have any wheels on it." They took us to a field at the bottom of the estate where pushed well into the field was our beloved car on blocks fully stripped out, devoid of car radio, wheels and tyres and personal items. Tony towed our caravan (we followed behind in our second vehicle) to our holiday and he subsequently came back to return us home.

Early September 1992 we discovered, excitingly, that Carol was pregnant again.

Good progress was being had at work to such a degree that my boss wanted me to temporarily manage the larger Blackburn branch for the crucial Christmas period starting November 1992 until January 1993. So it was back on the road again leaving Carol (pregnant) and the two boys and two dogs at home (déjà vu). This meant hotel living yet again and commuting across the Pennines on the notorious A66 to the M6 in the depths of winter. For my first day at the store I set off on the Sunday evening so that I could start early at 6.30am Monday and meet the early morning staff receiving the days goods and make a good first impression. Well what a lasting impression that turned out to be.

As I am not a very good packer Carol always excellently packed for me. So my new dark blue pin-striped suit was packed and placed into the car. It was a Sunday night so I was travelling casually. When I got to the hotel and unpacked it soon became apparent that I did not have my black leather work shoes! A quick call home confirmed that Carol couldn't remember packing them; she even offered to drive down with them but of course I couldn't let her do that.

So what was to be the strategy for the next day, should I go in later after the shops had opened and I could buy some shoes before work or still proceed as planned? Anyway my decision was to stick with the original plan. So at 6.30am Monday morning I turned up in my dark blue pin-striped suit with new white trainers, and introduced myself as their new manager. What a picture. They didn't say anything at the time but for many years afterwards I kept being reminded.

The travelling at times was tricky as often the snow gates were shut on the A66 and I had to make the circuitous trip using the A1 detouring through Ripon and Harrogate. I didn't make it home every weekend, but on those occasions the company paid for Carol and the kids to travel down and stop with me in the hotel. The kids thought it was great using the hotel pool and facilities.

Anyway we had a very successful Christmas trading period and mid-January 1993 I returned to "Bishop". By mid-march 1993 I was promoted to manager of the Durham store, which did not require a move of house this time as I could easily commute daily. The remit given was to prepare the store for a major refit as part of a major company trial and to make a success of it. Only ten stores in the company were to be in the trial that would involve regular feedback to the executive directors in person at our Nottingham Head Office. The trial (titled "Superstretch") was in each of the large department-like stores to remove inventory ranges such as Audio and Cookshop and to massively increase the space given to the Toiletries and Healthcare ranges and determine the effect on customer footfall, sales and most importantly profit.

The Durham store was situated in the historic market place in the absolute centre of Durham city and it was an absolute pleasure, at lunchtime, to walk around and sit by the river, admiring both castle and cathedral.

Durham is an UNESCO World Heritage Site (listed in 1986 and consisting of Durham Cathedral, Durham Castle and the buildings located between them).

Durham Cathedral (classed as one of Europe's great medieval buildings and one of the finest examples of Norman architecture) was built between 1093 and 1133. It contains the shrines of two Saints, Bede and Cuthbert. The venerable Bede lived in the seventh century and is considered "the Father of English history". St Cuthbert was instrumental in spreading Christianity in the North of England. The cathedral has been attracting pilgrims (and still does to this day) for over 900 years.

Durham Castle's construction began in 1072 under the orders of William the Conqueror, and this construction was supervised by the Earl of Northumberland until he was executed in 1076 for rebelling against William. The castle then came under the control of the Bishop of Durham (named Walcher, who purchased the earldom and became the first of the Prince-Bishops of Durham).

The castle was of strategic importance both to defend the troublesome border with Scotland as well as to control local English rebellions and invading Danes. A Prince-Bishop had the right to raise an army, mint his own coins and levy taxes. As long as he remained loyal to the King of England he could govern as a virtually autonomous ruler, reaping the revenue from his territory, but remaining mindful of his role of protecting England's Northern frontier. In 1832 Durham Castle ceased being the Bishop's palace and residence as that became Auckland Castle (Bishop Auckland).

Durham Castle was then donated to the University of Durham by Bishop Van Mildert. Durham University is a collegiate public research university and described as the third-oldest university in England (after Oxford and Cambridge). It has 17 colleges mainly scattered around the city centre.

I like my history but the relevance of all this in retailing terms means catering for the needs of students, tourists and visitors (from all over the world).

Also located close to the city centre is HM Prison Durham (built in 1816) which on visiting days unfortunately brought in another kind of tourist and we had to increase our store detective contingent as shoplifting was more prevalent on those days.

Durham used to be a category A, 600 cell prison for men and women) and former inmates included (to name but a few), Mary Ann Cotton, Myra Hindley, Ian Brady, Rosemary West and Ronald Kray: quite a list of notoriety. Durham is currently a reception prison for remand adult/young male prisoners divided with seven wings spanning secure units, plus a segregation and healthcare section, mainly serving the courts of County Durham, Tyne and Wear, Teeside and Cumbria.

Chapter 9

Our Ross

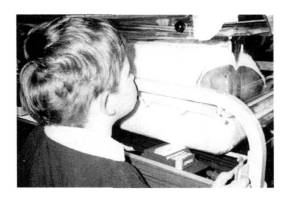

On Tuesday May 4th (Star Wars Day) 1993 I was out with our good friend and neighbour at the pub quiz in the "Top House", Canney (pronounced "Can-Ee") Hill. As it was three weeks before the baby's due arrival date I had hired a "pager" (no mobile phones then) so that I could be urgently contacted when there was any news.

I then had a message from the pub landlady (whom Carol had telephoned) to urgently contact her. At around about the same time my pager pinged with the message "waters broken come home". And so in a "mad dash" I drove home.

At home we then contacted Bishop Auckland Maternity Unit who informed us that as the waters had broken they would send an ambulance. Sister-in-laws and mother-in-law were contacted (who were on standby to take care of Lewis and Sean). Panic and concern then set in as Carol was taken by ambulance. I followed in our car once the family had arrived. Carol was admitted to the delivery suite and I remained with her for several hours until, again, I was told to go home as nothing was happening for a few hours (déjà vu)!

I went home to check that the boys were ok and then returned to the hospital at around 9am, as I had not heard from the hospital. Carol said her contractions had started and had informed the maternity staff of this fact and yet they seemed dismissive of it (despite Carol having two previous births and so therefore being an experienced, and not a new, mother) and they started to "induce" with an IV drip. What subsequently followed was an extremely painful labour (for which she was administered Pethidine), and I felt so helpless. At 2.55pm, 5th May 1993 our perfectly and fully formed and crying son Ross Jordan Atkinson was born (weight 3120g). Shortly after which Ross was whisked away in a baby incubator to the specialist baby unit, with the words "precautionary" and "he's going to be alright". Carol was still in complete shock and pain and was "wheel-chaired" into the shower to clean up. I was also in utter shock and could neither believe nor comprehend what (or why) this was happening.

They brought Ross to Carol for feeding and she instinctively knew something was wrong and told the midwife that Ross looked very pale (grey even) and was having difficulty breathing and feeding and asked could the doctor be called.

To our dismay the midwife appeared to be dismissive of this and didn't seem or want to listen to an experienced mother, and baby Ross was again whisked away. We then had a wait of several hours (an eternity it seemed) until we were then told that there was no Paediatrician on site (as it was a midwife-led unit) and that they had paged the doctor. Another what-felt extremely prolonged period of time elapsed (how long was so difficult to say in our state of shock and bewilderment). When she eventually arrived, the Paediatrician told us that Ross was very poorly and they would conduct "further" tests.

Several hours later a nurse told us to "fear the worst" in that Ross might not make it through the night and did we want to arrange for him to be baptised. Carol regularly attended, with the boys, Sunday school and Sunday service at Woodhouse Close Church and the Reverend Peter Sinclair was able to come to the maternity unit mid-evening and he very kindly baptised Our Ross. One of the special baby care unit nurses had just returned from a trip to Israel and had brought home a vial of water from the River Jordan and she donated it to us as it seemed appropriate for the baptism.

After the baptism we tried to get some rest and the hospital had a single bed that Carol and I could use overnight as Ross was so poorly. Of course sleep couldn't manifest itself and we spent our second night awake worrying and worrying. Sometime, around 6 or 7am, another consultant came to see us. He explained that Ross needed to be transferred to the Royal Victoria Hospital, Newcastle upon Tyne, for standard treatment in a specialist ventilator. He also said that there was a possibility that Ross could be entered into a specialist trial called ECMO which might give his lungs a better chance to recover from the Group B Streptococcus infection that was causing his difficulty with survival. Every parent wants to do the best for their child, no matter what and this was certainly the case and so we agreed to go for the trial.

As it was a trial Ross had to be "selected" randomly by a computer as to whether it would be standard ventilation at the RVI or ECMO at the Freeman Hospital Newcastle. Of course as a pharmacist I clearly understood the case for randomised drug trials but this was a "different kettle of fish" and it concerned the life or death of our child. There was again an indeterminable wait whilst this was decided, and we just became acutely anxious and worried "zombies" which was a state in which we were to exist for some time to come. The decision was in Ross's favour and so preparations were made for a travel ventilator, specialist ambulance (under blue emergency sirens) and nursing team to take Ross to the Freeman and we followed in our car.

ECMO (ExtraCorporeal Membrane Oxygenation) is described as "an extracorporeal technique of providing prolonged cardiac and respiratory support to persons whose heart and lungs are unable to provide an adequate amount of gas exchange or perfusion to sustain life". The technology is largely derived from cardiopulmonary bypass and uses a device called a membrane oxygenator (artificial lung).

Its aim is "to keep the body going" allowing the lungs and body to fight an infection. In 1993 it was in its early stages especially in paediatrics, hence the trial.

It has very recently come to the "public fore" during the Covid 19 pandemic.

During our wait to transfer, my dad contacted his niece's husband (who was a Senior Cardio-Thoracic Surgeon at the Freeman) to let him know the situation. Fortunately he was on hand at the Freeman and was able to assist when Ross had a cardiac arrest on arrival and exchange. Ross was then taken to theatre and the ECMO started, Ross was then placed in baby intensive care in the Children's Heart Unit Freeman Hospital (CHUF).

When we were allowed into the unit and saw that Ross was splayed out on a specialist table (bed) with what seemed like dozens and dozens of tubes and lines going in and out of his body. It looked like something from a horror movie and we were all living that horror, something you would never wish on your worst enemy (not that we have any). "Why us?"

Carol by this time had started to bleed heavily again and was admitted to a ward at the hospital and because of Ross's situation she was allowed to stay at the hospital which enabled her to visit Ross whenever she was allowed (it was a very specialist ICU with three ECMO beds and only one set of parents allowed in at any one time).

So it was with a heavy heart that each night I left Carol and Ross at the hospital and travelled home to Bishop Auckland and spent time with our beautiful children, Lewis and Sean, who were being well looked after by family during the day.

At the onset of ECMO we were told that it was only for ten days as any longer than that was likely to be unsurvivable.

For the next ten days we lived traumatised in a "Zombie-like" state of existence and in limbo, trying to "keep strong" for each other and the boys hoping and praying for Ross's recovery. During this time close family were also allowed to visit Carol and Ross, for which we were very grateful.

On around May 13th consultants enlightened us as to their findings of the latest scan and tests they had just completed.

We were then told that the scans and brain stem tests showed extensive brain damage and that if Ross survived the ECMO that he would in all likelihood be quadriplegic, deaf, dumb and blind and that that "would be no existence" and also unfair to our boys. They recommended switching off Ross's life support, what a shock and a hard place to be!

They then told us to go home and talk it over with the rest of the family. Another very troubled evening for us and what a decision that nonetheless had to be made. How could we make a decision to turn off the life support of our baby Ross whom Carol had carried to full term? An impossible dilemma for us both. After many tears and much soul searching together, we made the decision to switch off the life support following the termination of the ECMO and so we returned the next day to the Freeman, with such apprehension and heavy hearts.

The doctors did some final tests and the ECMO and life support were switched off and Ross placed into our arms in which at 7pm **14th May** 1993 he sadly died (exactly one year to the date of our miscarriage, so heart wrenching). Despite the circumstances it was lovely to be able to hold him in our arms, he will always be loved, remembered and never forgotten. We then returned home and told our family and gave many a hug and kiss to Lewis and Sean.

The nursing and medical team at CHUF were exceptional and so empathetic, as were the chaplaincy support team. A welfare worker member of the chaplaincy team supported and accompanied (in fact drove me on May 17th) to the registration office in Newcastle city centre to register Ross's death. (Death certificate giving cause of death as Respiratory Distress Syndrome, Cardiovascular collapse and Cerebral damage.)

We had been asked permission for a post mortem to be carried out but we declined as we thought that Ross had been operated on enough and couldn't bear the thought of him being cut up on a mortuary slab. Was this decision correct? We most definitely agreed at the time that it was.

Another difficult task I faced was to register Ross's birth, which had to be done at Bishop Auckland, the following day. We also had to engage a funeral director and arrange a funeral. The latter was arranged with the fantastic support of close family and close friends without whose help we don't know how it would have happened or how we would have got through it.

My mam and dad were so distraught at our loss, it must have reminded them so much of the loss of my brother David, something which they never discussed. Unfortunately my dad and I share the same fate in that we had both lost a dear son and brother, life can be so cruel.

The funeral director was also brilliant in that he arranged collection of Ross from the hospital and interred him in his funeral parlour. Carol wanted to visit Ross in the parlour. I was reluctant to do so, as I had said my goodbyes at the hospital, and yet I needed to help and support Carol so we both went together. The director had advised us against cremation as he said that in such young babies the bones are so soft that after cremation there is little or no ashes and so a burial was arranged at Bishop Auckland Town Cemetery (the funeral service was to be held at Woodhouse Close Church, conducted by Rev. P. Sinclair).

On the day of the funeral, which was attended by a vast number of family, friends and work colleagues from far and wide, we were unbelievably grateful for so much love, compassion and support shown by so many. We had also made the decision to fully include Lewis and Sean with the whole funeral as we felt it was so important for them to not to be bewildered by all the tears and people and to share all our love.

My glass (measure), normally always half full had a massive crack in it and was completely empty and devoid of content and somehow needed repair and refilling.

The "emotional cycle of change" illustrates that when a life-changing event occurs you have to fall over the proverbial precipice and into the deepest part of the trough hopefully to rise out of the trough and into a better (higher) place than when you fell in. At this point we were well into the deepest place but determined to climb out with love and support for each other and the boys and with help from family and friends and I am glad to say that we did.

Several weeks after the funeral, the consultant from Bishop Auckland Maternity Unit asked us to come in for a review, which on reflection seemed to be for their benefit rather than ours, at which they discussed the cause as Group B Streptococcal (GBS) infection. Regretfully no counselling was offered and yet this would have been so beneficial.

Streptococcus is a commensal bacterium that lives in the nasopharynx and forms part of the natural bacteria flora in the body of men and women. It can invade (colonise) the rest of the body in very old and very young people resulting in pneumonia, sepsis and meningitis.

Commensal bacteria act on the host's immune system to induce protective responses that prevent colonisation and invasion by pathogens. GBS is also a common bacterium which is carried in the vagina and rectum of two to four in ten women (20–40%) and is not harmful but it can affect a baby at around the time of birth and occasionally cause serious infection in newborn babies, and very rarely during pregnancy and before labour. The risk is extremely small and happens in about one in 1750 pregnancies. Statistics show that between 1981 and 1996, in Britain, there were 51 neonatal deaths (where GBS was the prime cause) out of a total of 630,206 livebirths. But of course just one is too many and devastating for any parent.

In fact as far back as 1992 America issued the first formal screening and treatment guidelines for GBS in pregnancy but it has taken the UK many years (and perhaps many preventable deaths) to implement. In fact in 2003 the NHS only issued "risk-based guidelines". However, this stance eventually changed and the UK screening rate improved from 42% in 2014 to 75% in 2015 and 98% of women accepted the offer of screening. This is not the full story as on October 2021 a new major clinical trial began (led by experts at the University of Nottingham) which is the first in the world to measure the effectiveness of two tests to identify group B strep bacteria in late pregnancy or labour, compared with the approach of identifying pregnant women with "risk factors" for their newborn developing the infection. So this small risk is still "out there" and I wholeheartedly recommend that all pregnant women discuss GBS with their clinicians during the latter third of their pregnancy.

We will always question "what if" i.e.

- What if the staff had listened to Carol?
- What if the labour was allowed to progress naturally and the extreme labour not compounded by IV induction?
- What if the staff had called the doctor /consultant earlier?
- What if the birth had taken place in another hospital?

Questions that can never now be answered. They say that time is a great healer, which of course it is, and yet there have been many an occasion and articles in the news as recently as August 2022 (time of writing) which cause us both to relive the trauma. I name just a few examples of recent enquiries that have filled our TV screens and our minds.

- 2013 Morecambe Bay NHS Foundation Trust enquiry reporting that the deaths of 11 babies and one mother at Furness General Hospital were avoidable and a result of a "lethal mix" of failings. Amongst the findings were that the maternity unit had been "dysfunctional" with "substandard care" provided by staff "deficient in skills and knowledge".

- 2022 Shrewsbury and Telford Hospital NHS report reporting on the failure that led to the deaths of 200 babies and nine mothers and a corresponding "Ockenden" enquiry and report.

- Nottingham University NHS Trust press expose that between 2010 and 2020 46 babies had suffered brain damage and 19 stillborn in the Trust maternity units now subject to another "Ockenden" enquiry and report.

Clearly, in my opinion, across the country there has been a national systemic failure in maternity provision leadership which is not to criticise the majority of the dedicated maternity staff teams.

We were so upset by these recent reports that I wrote to the Ockenden Maternity Review Team highlighting Our Ross's story and experience, as somehow the dots needed to be joined between all these events.

An extract of their reply follows. *"I am sorry that the recent coverage of our report publication has caused distress to you and your family. Due to the passage of time it is likely that the maternity records for your wife will have been destroyed so it would be difficult to follow this up. That said you could contact the PALS department at the Trust and raise your concerns with them, they should be able to advise you how best to proceed.*

"I am sorry that I cannot be of much more help and I wish you well in getting the answers you seek."

A very well-intentioned and empathetic reply. I know in my heart it is too late but it was important to let them know that many couples over many years have been affected by such traumatic circumstances.

*

We visit Ross's grave several times a year (and have done since 1993 to the present day, 2022) but at least twice a year: once around his birthday/loss and once at Christmas to leave a little gift and say a little prayer and let him know that we love him and that he is forever loved. It is more difficult now and during my illness and also as we now live in Lancashire (more of which later in this story). Whenever we visit the graveside (which is situated in a special area reserved for children) we are also reminded, by the dozens of child and baby graves present, that many a couple in Bishop Auckland have also suffered such loss. Every October (except during Covid lockdowns) the CHUF chaplaincy hold a remembrance memorial (which we attend) at Heaton in Newcastle for all the children lost every year in the Children's heart unit. Hymns are sung, prayers given, and a candle lit and name read aloud for every child. It is very humbling and thought provoking as the number is now so large. When on holiday either at home or abroad whenever we visit a church or cathedral we always light a candle for him.

There are some songs that are particularly poignant for me. One is "Tears in Heaven" by Eric Clapton (written as a memorial for his four-year-old son's tragic loss). A song that I would later learn to play on my acoustic guitar.

Later around September 1993 I attended a Boots Christmas Conference at which they played the latest Boots advert which was accompanied by a video supporting the company's latest charity to support, which was Children In Need and for whom funds were raised for by selling Christmas reindeer antlers.

The video showed very moving images of children with various physical disabilities being happy and looked after in the care of their family and friends. The accompanying soundtrack was "Drive" by The Cars. It made me think of Ross and I sat quietly in the auditorium silently crying to myself. I also had to leave the room to compose myself for five minutes. The lyrics still move me and remind me of Our Ross to this day.

After the funeral it was time to pick ourselves up and to try and get back to our "normal" lives for the well-being of us all as a family. We enjoyed our holidays with the boys and good fun times and with family and friends creating such fond memories. Our good neighbour (who was General Manager of Eaton Yale in Bolton which had a sister factory in Pamplona, Spain) asked us if we could "take in" a Spanish au pair for the summer. He had been asked by his secretary, in Pamplona, if her daughter could come across and stay the summer to help improve her English. Unfortunately he was going through a divorce at the time and living at home with his two teenage sons (with their raging hormones) and so thought that it might not be such a good idea to have a teenage Spanish girl staying with them so he asked us to.

So she came to say with us for the summers of '93 and '94. "Au pair" is not the correct description as we treated her like a member of our family and she accompanied us at all family occasions and weekend trips away. We also acted as tourist guides showing her the delights of County Durham, North Yorkshire and Cumbria. She was a great help and support for Carol at such a difficult time for the family and the boys loved her, though four-year-old Sean regularly tormented her by hanging from the rear pockets of her denim jeans to much hilarity. The last we heard from her was that she had married a professional Spanish footballer back in her home country.

Chapter 10

The Cat Burglars

I returned to work straight after the weekend following the funeral as the refit and "superstretch trial" was to begin within the week.

One night in the early hours I received a telephone call from my distressed assistant manager who had been "called out" in response to the alarm being triggered. As he was local he attended promptly and unlocked the store and entered to check what had "set off" the alarm and went up to the second floor sales area when he observed a pair of legs sticking out of the ceiling!

The attempted burglar was rapidly making their exit through the air vent they had entered (via cutting through the aluminium ducting on the roof). Fortunately they had "legged it" and been intercepted before they had managed to steal anything. This was not the last time that the store was burgled.

The refit and trial lasted a full 12 months (to measure the effect on the stores Trading Account), and was very tiring and intensive involving many a late night and weekend working and as such kept me busy and focussed. It resulted in "lost" sales from "lost" inventories exceeding the sales and profit budgets set and was the best performing of the ten selected stores. I had to present to the directors the reasons for our success (which did no harm at all to my profile with senior management). The company learnt much from such a trial which helped focus its future strategy to focus on Health and Beauty.

Carol during this time was undertaking voluntary

work at Woodhouse playgroup and as a parent governor at Aclet Nursery School whilst juggling looking after Lewis and Sean.

During the autumn of '94 I was asked to temporarily manage the Sunderland city centre store whilst my fellow colleague had some minor surgery. Of course this did not involve a move but did involve a busy commute between "Bishop" and Sunderland and following this I returned to my Durham store.

It was November again, the time of the year that police told me was the month of the cat burglars (presumably thieving "to order" for Christmas). As I arrived very early one morning, upon opening the store I noticed some items scattered on the sales floor (indeed medicine boxes). Then to my horror I looked into the dispensary and there was a massive gaping hole between the dispensary shelving open to the outside world at the rear of the store some 15 feet plus above ground level. The store was built on a slope with the front entrance level with the market square but the rear of the store ground level was 20 feet or so below that of the front.

The dispensary was completely wrecked and hundreds of packets of medicines stolen, especially those medicines which could be classed as addictive and had a "street" value and corresponding market. The Controlled Drugs cabinet (of "golden key" fame) was intact as it was alarmed. The thieves obviously knew what they "were about" as opening this would immediately trigger an alarm direct to the local police station and a rapid response. I then telephoned the police and whilst waiting for the Scenes of Crimes investigators I proceeded up the central staircase to the first floor which was the location of our Beauty Hall, Photographic and Baby Departments.

More devastation confronted me in that shelves had been completely stripped of stock and discarded stock was scattered everywhere. Every camera, every bottle of expensive fine fragrance, hundreds and hundreds of premium cosmetics, including Boots No.7 and No.17 ranges, baby clothes and equipment had been taken. We estimated that at least £250,000 of stock had been taken (we were jammed to the rafters with stock for the busy Christmas trading period).

It appeared like they had been able to spend hours and hours in the store without triggering an alarm. Every door in the building was alarmed so they had gained entry and exit without activation and they had destroyed the CCTV cameras. Front and rear, outside CCTV cameras had been broken or spray painted over. Where they had sledge-hammered the bricks in the dispensary wall was (unknown to me and store staff) apparently an old window which had been bricked up. The store had been well "cased" for the job. Was it just a coincidence that it was a period of time just after a major refit?

We had to shut the store for a couple of days (24 hours for the police) and another 24 hours to repair as much as possible and restock. Head Office put in place an emergency plan and contractors were quickly sent for. Head Office warehouses sent emergency stock on specially arranged transport and local surrounding stores asked to donate as much Christmas specific stock as possible and extra staffing was arranged. A miracle at Christmas in logistical terms.

So after 48 hours we were open and ready for our busy Christmas trading period.

A few days later the police informed us that in West Yorkshire a routine car stop had been made revealing cameras and fragrance in the car boot and arrests weremade. The cameras were attributed to our store via their serial numbers as we still had the boxes and instructions (with numbers) to those cameras, because they formed part of the "live displays" and said boxes were safely stored in the stockroom. Police intelligence informed us that the burglary had been committed by a local gang (from a local estate) for a criminal gang in West Yorkshire where it was also to be "fenced". Only a tiny proportion of stock was recovered.

Despite this, and due to the brilliant efforts of all my staff, we had a reasonably successful Christmas in sales and footfall terms. Profits were of course down due to recovery and staffing costs.

Well January soon came round and I was on the move again! I had been asked to temporarily manage the larger Bolton city centre store (perhaps I was being used as a trouble shooter), which meant travelling the A66 and M6 yet again and staying away in Bolton Hotels, much to Carol's delight I'm sure. The boys did enjoy spending the odd weekend away with me in a hotel again.

One particular weekend journey home springs to mind. As I was exiting the M6 at Tebay heavy snow began to fall with a strong wind blowing the snow horizontally in my windscreen's field of view.

It got so heavy and thick that it was a "white out" and driving conditions were almost impossible and dangerous and so I crawled into Brough, but the flashing warning signs were informing me that the A66 was closed and the snow gates shut. I was desperate to get home to Carol and the boys and so foolheartedly decided to take the B6276 road, up over the moors to Middleton-Teesdale (a road without snow gates and so could be blocked by the weather).

Coming out of Brough on this road (for any budding Ordnance Survey map readers) there is a very steep hill with a bend at "Intake Side" where about a dozen cars were abandoned part way up.

I thought "Do I go for it?"

"Bulled" by the fact I had a shovel in the boot, I did. I was driving a white Ford Sierra estate with rear wheel drive, not the best vehicle to make such an attempt. The car slewed 45 degrees across the road and inch by inch (like a crab on the beach or like a sidewinder snake) kept on going, past the abandoned cars and made it to the top (it took nearly an hour to edge up that half mile).

Then I was on top of the moors and about a mile further up at "Windmore End" near a cattle grid I could just about "make out" a huge wall of snow. As I approached it, to my relief, a tractor had just punched a hole through it. I eventually made it to Middleton-Teesdale, where I took the B6282 to Bishop Auckland and made it, very late, to the sanctuary of home, tired and with a sheer sense of relief for both Carol and myself (it was still snowing!). A feat I would never attempt to repeat.

The next day I was speaking with my neighbour (who was also returning from his Bolton factory) and discovered that he did not make it home. He had abandoned his car and along with others slept on the floor of a local pub, just before the town of Brough. I grinned with satisfaction that I had managed to get home.

I returned to the Durham store in April but I soon found myself on the "promotion list" again. In July I found myself being interviewed for the permanent management position of the larger Blackburn Store. Prior to this I had to produce a business plan of the store to include a SWOT (strengths, weaknesses, opportunities and threats) analysis of the store, a full personal review of key staff and a competitor analysis together with my list of priorities for my first year! The interviewing Area Manager then conducted a full competence-based interview and then dissected my business plan (just like the TV show *The Apprentice*).

Immediately after the interview he said that I had got the job but would I like to be appointed the manager of the even larger Lancaster store instead (a better promotion in a nicer location). I said yes straight away (as I was delighted) and he said, "Perhaps you'd better phone Carol first", which of course I did and she was delighted too. On 3rd August 1995 I started in Lancaster and we were on the move again and the house was for sale.

Chapter 11

Lancaster

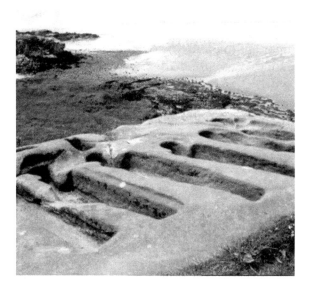

Just a little snippet about the historic city of Lancaster, which in many ways has symmetry with Durham in that it has a castle above a river (Lune), a cathedral, a university and a prison. Also, like Durham, most of the land in the area is either owned by the church, the university or the Crown (in this case the Duchy of Lancaster, Her Majesty the Queen).

There was a third century Roman fort with bath house upon which in the 13th Century Lancaster Castle was built. This was besieged by Robert the Bruce around 1322 (who burnt the town) but although the castle was damaged it resisted the attack and was then restored by

John of Gaunt.

Lancaster Castle became an Assizes (courts and prison) and in 1612 it was infamously known as the site of the Pendle witch trials. Lancaster earned the nickname, "the Hanging Town" as it sentenced more people to be hanged than any other in the country outside London.

The Port of Lancaster (St George's Quay) in the 18th Century became one of the UK's busiest and the fourth most important in the UK slave trade. However its role as a major port was curtailed as the river began to silt up. Morecambe, Glasson Dock and Sunderland Point became outposts for a short period of time. Nearby Heysham is now a freight port, but Glasson Dock remains a port for fertiliser and grain. Because of this Lancaster is mainly a "service" trading city for grain, textiles, chemicals, livestock, paper, synthetic and mineral fibres and farm machinery. High-tech industries are now emerging particularly under the influence of the university.

I was, again, staying in a hotel for several months (more fun for the boys) whilst looking for a new home (literally, as we were to buy a new build). The major difference, this time, was that we had to find a school for the boys (Lewis about to enter Year Two and Sean Year One). To this end, as it was summer and school holidays, Carol brought the caravan down and we stayed on a campsite in Glasson Dock (together with Carol's mam and dad in their van to help look after the boys).

Whilst we were staying Carol took us on a day trip out to visit Half Moon Bay in Heysham, a place of fond childhood memories for her of lazy beach days, camping with her family. She was extolling its virtues and directing me to the car park that she could remember when a great monstrosity loomed into our vision. Someone had decided to build a huge concrete block of a nuclear power station. It dominated the area, the horizon and glorious views across Morecambe Bay for many miles around in this idyllic location. (Heysham One was commissioned in 1983, and Heysham Two in 1988.)

Despite this Heysham village remains very quaint with picturesque walks and historical buildings. Near St Patrick's Chapel you can find the "barrows" consisting of six rock-cut graves which are thought to be some of the earliest examples of Christian burials in the country. Estimated to be from around the 11th century, each grave being hewn from solid rock and because a large number of bones were found (including a child grave), it is thought that such graves were a reliquary and were reserved for the privileged.

Six graves in total are present and four are clearly body shaped with holes at the edge where a wooden cross would have stood. The heavy rain experienced in the North West often fills these graves but what interests me the most (as a fan of their music) is that Black Sabbath featured these (in black and white) as an album cover for *The Best of Black Sabbath*. I have taken photographs of these graves to try and replicate the album cover.

It was difficult to find a primary school in Lancaster that could start both boys at the end of October half-term and so we cast our net further and settled on the lovely market town of Garstang (where we still live today). The boys then attended Garstang County Primary School and then later Garstang High School.

Garstang is an ancient market town ten miles south of Lancaster and ten miles north of Preston. It is overlooked by the ruined remains of Greenhalgh Castle built in 1490. The castle was, during the English Civil War, one of the last two Royalist strongholds in Lancashire to succumb to Oliver Cromwell's forces in 1644/45 after which demolition teams were sent in to prevent it being used again for military purposes. Garstang was granted market status in the early 1300s and it still markets on a Thursday to this day. The town has a strong sense of community values and because of this celebrates an arts festival, agricultural show, steam and games fair and a children's festival to name a few.

Garstang, in 2000, became "the world's first Fairtrade Town", influencing many towns, cities and cons around the UK towards the "Fairtrade" principles.

Geographically it lays on the River Wyre, River Calder, and the Lancaster Canal close to the A6 and M6 roads and the West Coast Mainline. It is also in the foothills of the Forest of Bowland, an AONB (Area of Outstanding Natural Beauty), all in all a lovely place to settle.

On moving to Lancaster we became active members of Lancaster Volleyball Club (which I served as player coach and treasurer) and as such gained many new friends.

I was to remain as manager of Boots Lancaster (initially with around 100 staff to be responsible for) for nine years until 2003. During which time there were many happy events that "spring" to mind.

One such occasion was 5th September 1997, Princess Dianna's funeral, the date of which I am sure many will remember where they were at the time. I was at work, but many companies had given their staff time off to share in the mourning of her passing and to watch her funeral on TV. We closed for half a day but as a pharmacy, under our NHS contract terms, we had to still provide a dispensing service. As such we kept the pharmacy and dispensary open, with the rest of the store partitioned off. It was manned by myself and two volunteer dispensers.

I brought a portable TV from home and set it up on the counter for my staff and any customer/patient who may avail us of our services, nobody did for the whole two hours it was on. It was so surreal. Lancaster city centre is compact and encircled by a one-way road system bounded by the River Lune, and is normally extremely busy but during this time period the roads were deserted as was the shopping centre. This was never to be repeated during my time at work, but it happened during the recent Covid 19 pandemic and subsequent lockdowns.

With my promotion to Lancaster my remuneration package included a "company car" for the first time and we had to choose from a designated list. The car I chose was a Citroen Xantia because it had 129ydropneumatics self-levelling suspension which was very useful to tow our caravan. The car was also used at times to deliver oxygen and medicines to nursing homes, which helped for tax purposes to increase my "company mileage". The latter tax arrangements were, at the time, quite ludicrous and resulted in us senior store managers driving separately to the same meetings to record company mileage to offset the tax burden. At that time climate change was not the dominant story it is now.

I had this car for about two and a half years until I wrote it off. I was on the promotion list again and on my way to an interview for the hub management of all the York city centre stores – I didn't quite get there. I was travelling, from Lancaster, across and over the Trough of Bowland, on a very twisty road, (the A65 via Blubberhouses) listening to a leadership training meeting, when near a bend I glanced and saw a "give way sign" and thought this was on a side road and didn't apply to me. How wrong I was. I overshot a junction and ploughed the car under the side of an articulated lorry, crash, bang wallop. Fortunately, the lorry had side bars that brought my car to an abrupt stop and momentarily, just before the airbags exploded, I saw the car bonnet fly off and the car battery fly into the air. Fortunately no other vehicle was involved and the lorry driver and myself were both unhurt (except my pride). The lorry was unscathed too but my Xantia was a write-off and blocking this main road in both directions. The police arrived at the scene but they were non-plussed to be there as they were an armed response crew and I was bundled into the back of their vehicle tight up against their sealed central rifle and arms cabinet. They redirected the traffic around the grassy banks until the breakdown truck arrived.

The truck then towed me to the nearest garage, which fortunately allowed me use of their phone. I then called my interviewer and my area office to make arrangements to recover the vehicle. I was informed that arrangements did not cover the driver. So in a state of shock, I had to arrange a hire car myself and then drive home. A few weeks later I was interviewed and didn't get the position. I guess the stars were aligned against it.

In September 1998, I was asked to participate in a company pilot scheme and was appointed Regional Professional Development Manager. This job was to move me away from grass roots pharmacy and into a strategic "ivory tower" role. This was based at the Northern Regional Office in Eldon Square, Newcastle upon Tyne and involved a commute from Garstang up the M6 and across the A66 again (in the reverse direction this time but again in the winter months) and meant staying away in Newcastle hotels.

The area this position covered was the whole of Cumbria and Northumberland (up to the Scottish borders) and all of Lancashire. The regional area also took in the whole of Scotland but as Scottish pharmacy law differs from that of England and Wales that was covered by a Scottish pharmacist colleague reporting to the same Regional Manager.

My role was to drive the healthcare and dispensing businesses (for which I had a line reporting function to Head Office) and to ensure pharmacy operational, professional and training standards were being met.

Externally it was to liaise (and ultimately influence) a retail Pharmacy Agenda within the government Health Action Zones, Health Authorities and Local Pharmaceutical Committees. For example one of the areas we were developing was the early implementation of NHS Direct (later to become NHS111). And I thought I wasn't political!

Anyway with all the travelling, being away from home and family and missing the pharmacy coal face as well as patient interaction I decided that this was not for me and agreed a return to Lancaster.

Back at store the local Lancaster Drug Dependency Unit had decided to stop its dispensing function and concentrate solely on medical prescribing and social counselling. We were asked to provide a dispensing service for methadone and other opiate replacement therapies. This was a dilemma for me because as a pharmacist it was the correct health promotion path but as a store manager my concern was both for my customers and staff as, unfortunately, some (a minority) of the DDU patients were of the most deprived and addicted kind who had been excluded from the store for shoplifting.

If a person had been excluded from the store (which we were entitled to do as a private company) we had an obligation, under our NHS contract, to dispense any prescriptions presented by them. In these cases we would meet them at the door and then take their prescription for dispensing and then return with said prescription dispensed.

My professional side won and we took on dozens of their patients using formal agreed standards of behaviour to which they had to agree. Through my LPC role it was also agreed for other local pharmacies to participate.

It was satisfying to see those who made a success of the programme and "kicked" their addiction as they were "weened off" the methadone (opiate substitute) slowly. But unfortunately some fell by the wayside.

Within this time period the company employed an external consultant agency to deliver (with managerial support) a selling and customer service package for all staff to help us deliver a "competitive advantage".

This together with my self-development plans triggered a desire to learn further techniques and build upon current skills and tools to help "understand" people's motivation together with conflict and negotiation skills.

I consequently took an interest in personality profiling, (using Myers–Briggs), neurolinguistics programming (a model of human experience and communication) by reading *Frogs into Princes* by Richard Bandler, understanding that people have preferences about how they like to learn (Honey and Mumford's learning styles) and other personality testing methods such as Dr Porter's Relationship Awareness Training (personality typing in and out of conflict). All heavy brain-blowing (more about this later) stuff I guess but at the time I thought it would help me be a better leader. Who knows if that worked? But the pyscho-analysis would later be very useful.

Anyway in March 2000 I became manager of the two Morecambe stores as well as Lancaster and then in September 2001 I was asked to temporarily manage the Kendal and Windermere stores whilst providing additional support for the Cockermouth, Keswick, and Ambleside stores.

All this while retaining the "lead" on all pharmacy matters within Lancashire and The Lakes, which together with my past roles led to me being asked to represent the company LPCs and the Royal Pharmaceutical Society at the Labour Party Conference, 20th October 2002, at the Winter Gardens, Blackpool.

Prior to attending we had to be police vetted and have passes issued. Tony Blair (Prime Minister and Labour Party leader) was in attendance and he had invited his friend, former President of the USA (1993–2001) Bill Clinton to make a key note speech.

My role was to help "man" a display stand set up by a RPSGB Head Office member and to support them in promoting the role of pharmacy within the NHS, and to answer any delegates' or visiting dignitaries' questions. Also, to hand out the obligatory handouts of freebies and leaflets and a nice little miniature brass mortar and pestle. Tony and Bill did not visit me (their loss) but they, along with their entourage, could be seen in the distance.

Bill Clinton's speech included references to Iraq, Northern Ireland, September 11th, Kosovo and Africa etc. but for me the best part was his opening lines in which he drew attention to how much he had enjoyed the McDonald's in Blackpool, since he had never visited it before.

I can just imagine, in my mind's eye, the picture of American Secret Service agents surrounding McDonald's, Blackpool.

Oddly enough in Jan 2003 I was to temporarily (for three months) manage the Boots Blackpool store, a larger three-floored store with an external customer glass lift with views out to sea (our very own viewing platform). The Winter Gardens held many an event (not just political conferences) such as dance competitions, pigeon fanciers, keep-fit instructor's, dog grooming, rabbit keeping shows and weekends as well as musical events. A well-utilised venue with a very characterful interior décor and well worth a visit if ever in Blackpool (after all even Bill Clinton has visited).

During this period from 1996 onwards, Carol began to put her working career back on track and completed a "return to teaching certificate" which involved work experience at three Garstang primary schools as well as Devonshire Road Infants School in Blackpool (a very socially deprived and challenging area).

For a couple of years she also worked at the boys' school (Garstang County Primary) as a special care support assistant, helping a child with special educational needs.

In 1998 she joined Lancaster and Morecambe College to support and teach adults with severe learning difficulties, all roles which she had a particular empathy and skill set for and which she found very rewarding until she retired in 2018 (due to ill health).

It was around about this time that Carol, along with work colleagues, decided to abseil down the high rise building of Lancaster Teaching College in the name of charity (RNIB) for another work colleague who was blind and also taught in LMC's head injury department. It came to the day of reckoning and one by one all of her colleagues dropped out and did not participate.

However, Carol with steely determination, a "lot of bottle" and a desire not to disappoint either her blind colleague or the charity completed the task and raised "lots of eyebrows" and a significant amount of cash.

Chapter 12

A Broken Stick of Rock and the Clock

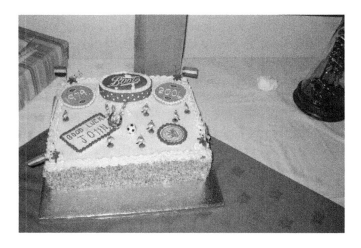

In January 2004 all senior Boots managers (my grade and above, including directors) were called to meetings around the country. At such meetings we were told that the company was restructuring and that around 50% of us would be made redundant and that we had to apply for new positions and attend a selection centre at Head Office. What a bombshell! Ironically the Director of Customer service who delivered this was a colleague, who all those years ago was on the leadership course (at Kegworth) with me and a participant in the "faked burst tyre ruse". He later went on to become CEO of the company.

I then had to arrive home and deliver the distressing news to Carol (we were so upset). My upset turned, internally, to anger and anguish asking how they could do this to us after so many years of loyal service. My Lancaster staff used to describe me as a stick of rock, which had the word "Boots" running through it. But now it was broken.

The selection centre (in Nottingham) was run by an independent agency (to avoid bias I guess) and involved us undertaking exam condition psychometric tests, a videoed interview and a presentation (for which you were given just one hour to prepare from the topic given on the day).

At my interview (competency based) the questioner asked, "What is the most difficult decision you have had to make?" To which I asked, "Do you mean inside or outside of work?" And his reply was "It makes no difference, just give me the most difficult." So I looked him straight in the eye (all that heavy psychology reading came to mind) and I said, "Turning off my son's life support machine, every other difficult decision 'pales' into insignificance when compared."

As you can probably imagine his face dropped, silence ensued and I guess he wished a hole could open and swallow him up. What an extremely stressful day for us all, after which I no longer wished to be part of the company (my pragmatic approach to life shining through).

A few weeks later I was informed that I had been successful at the selection centre and asked if I would like to accept a position managing ten stores in the Lakes area (for the same money) on a 12 month rolling contract! If not, then redundancy was offered (which it wouldn't be in 12 months' time if I wasn't successful in the new role). An intolerable decision but one which we had already made: I was leaving and taking redundancy. My boss and his boss (my RPDM boss) were also leaving. I had to work my full notice (no garden leave for me) and so on 1st July 2004 I left to turn full circle and return to grass roots pharmacy.

A few weeks previously I had been sent a letter, ironically from Head Office, asking me to select my 25-year award gift. I chose a skeleton clock with an upside down conical dome (reminding me of my conical glass measure now empty again).

My staff arranged a brilliant leaving party for me at the Garstang Country Hotel & Golf Club. Dress code was football shirts as they knew I was a keen Middlesbrough FC fan. It was a lovely party atmosphere with a disco and plenty of party food. Carol was, of course, invited (despite her Liverpool shirt) as she had attended all my staff functions over the years. My boss then proceeded with a slide presentation consisting of key photographs of both my early and Boots years (Carol had secretly provided them) and read out extracts from my company personal file. The DJ played some of my favourite music (not sure how "Sabbath Bloody Sabbath" was appreciated though). I was also presented with my clock (25 years service) and a print montage of Lancaster by the noted local artist *CHAZ*, flowers for Carol and other goodies. One of my staff had written and presented the following poem.

J.A. is leaving boots,
Where he has worked for twenty five years,
So if he is worried I will tell all his secrets,
Its time he realized his fears!

His long suffering wife called carol,
Has always competed with work,
But there are times in her life when she's wondered,
Did she really marry this berk!

Like the time she was in labour with Lewis,
John went on a slight detour,
So what if she's having a baby,
He had to take his keys to the store!

But long ago they were childhood sweethearts,
Although it wasn't love at first sight,
She called him "the posh boy from grammar",
But he must have got something right!

Coz she puts up with all his antics,
Although he often has her in a whirl,
Like the time he visited a restaurant,
Dressed up as his favourite "spice girl",

If it's a course he has to go on,
Carol always packs his case,
But she forgot to put his shoes in once,
Which left him with a red face?

All done up in his suit and tie,
The new bosses, he went to meet,
And he really made an impression that day,
With white trainers on his feet!

Now we all know john is sporty,
And supports "Middlesbrough FC"
He really wanted to play for them,
But luckily for them he's injured his knee!

You might prefer to forget his "other love"
As it involves a black rubber suit,
Not something to imagine behind dispensary,
On a wet Monday morning at boots!!

Johns other hobby is caravanning,
And he also likes heavy rock,
So he'll be happy listening to music,
While he sits and admires his "gold clock"!

We will all remember his party piece.
He likes to boogie to "tom",
He "struts his stuff" on the dance floor,
J.A is the original "sex bomb"!

As a boss we think he's served us well,
Although he's fondly known as "stress head",
But we've warned the staff in his new shop,
So now he is their, "problem" instead!

Seriously though john, all joking aside,
We wish you all the best,
As bosses come and bosses go,
You are better than the rest!!

All in all they had "done me proud" and had been a pleasure to work with, even when challenged with some difficult times. End of an era for me.

However, I had to move on. Using my contacts I was going to work for a pharmacist colleague and "run" a pharmacy he was buying, complete with premium fragrance and cosmetic business in Lytham. Unfortunately, the "due diligence" investigations threw up issues and he did not purchase and so I had no job.

I had a little time off to decide my option of being a self-employed locum pharmacist across Lancashire (again using my contacts).

The "time off" was to follow my son Lewis's school cycle ride from Land's End to John O'Groats. Carol was the support vehicle driver for the first leg (Land's End to Garstang, the mid-point).

For this point of the journey I travelled with Sean, in our family car, and we stayed at Trevella camping site in Newquay.

This location enabled us to see Lewis set off on his epic journey and Carol follow in the back up vehicle. As Sean was a keen carp fisherman and there being two lakes on site, we stayed in his "bivvy" whilst he fished. (He has subsequently become a proficient carper, and for any keen carp anglers out there his personal best carp is 51 pounds 4 ounces!) We also visited Fistral Beach for the surfing and bodyboarding. Lewis and school mates cycled back to Garstang and Carol handed over the support driver duties. Lewis then cycled to John O'Groats and Carol, Sean and I drove to meet him at the end (via Fort William, along Loch Ness to Inverness and then up through Wick). It was a very scenic drive but it must have been a tough cycle. We all then drove back home to Garstang, via Aviemore, Perth and Stirling.

It was then back to pharmacy, and work, for me and

Carol, as I undertook locum pharmacist duties for independents, and major multiples across Cumbria, Lancashire and Manchester. It was certainly a challenge especially experiencing clearly different standards of operation across the spectrum (an eye opener). After six months I decided that this was not for me and I became appointed Store Manager at the United Northwest Co-Operative flag ship store in Poulton-Le-Fylde.

It was here that I remained until my career came to an abrupt end in 2007/8 and the **patient** side of my "Patient Pharmacist" tale started to dominate.

Chapter 13

Do You Want the Good News First or the Bad News?

One evening (late December 2006) I left work to attend a local Co-Op area pharmacist/store manager meeting at the "Tickled Trout Hotel", Preston close to the M6, when in the car park I suddenly developed severe chest pains. I then telephoned Carol (my first thought rather than an ambulance as I should have done). She dashed from home and drove me to Preston Royal Infirmary A&E and immediately they put on oxygen, ECG and blood pressure monitoring etc. I was then kept in overnight for observation and tests.

In the middle of the night there must have been bed availability issues and I was transferred, via ambulance, to Chorley Hospital (little did I know that this was to become the start of my North West Hospital Grand Tour).

The following morning I was told that the "enzyme levels", which could show the presence of a heart attack, were clear. But that they wanted to run a "treadmill test in the cardiac unit". I was jogging gently on this treadmill, breathing through a spirometer (just like at University all those years ago) and, as they increased its speed, there was a look of alarm on the faces of the Technicians and they told me that it was too dangerous to continue and that I would need to see a cardiologist and have further tests (more cracks in the glass). I was then put on a suite of standard drugs to lower blood pressure, heart rate and cholesterol whilst waiting for a cardiologist appointment.

Fortunately, my remuneration package with the Co-Op

included private health care (they obviously wanted to take care of their managers to get them back to work ASAP). Very quickly I saw the cardiologist (in his private rooms) and he informed me that I needed to have an angiogram (in which a catheter and camera is inserted, via the wrist or thigh, up to the heart) to check for any blocked blood vessels in the muscle of the heart and if they found any they would there and then insert a "stent/s" to open any blocked vessels.

So it was off to Blackpool Victoria hospital this time for the procedure, fortunately for me no blockage was found. The cardiologist then arranged and conducted, at Preston hospital, an echocardiogram (basically an ultrasound scan of the heart, which checks the structure of the heart and assesses how the pumping chambers and valves are working). This assessment also indicated no major heart issues and only a slightly leaking heart valve, which apparently is common and doesn't cause any issues.

It was then decided and agreed to stop all the prescribed medications as my heart was, thankfully, ok and I could continue with work and playing volleyball (now for Garstang, as I had previously helped form the new club). What caused the chest pains was a mystery which can perhaps be explained shortly.

We then had a lovely Christmas time with friends and family.

Around early March 2007, I noticed that I was having hearing problems. I thought it was just age related but couldn't have been further wrong. I was visiting the Opticians for new glasses, and enquired if there were any hearing test appointments available. Luckily there were. The test indicated that I was profoundly deaf in the left ear and the technician immediately referred me to an ENT consultant, "Bravo" (it is from this stage that all my consultants will be assigned a phonetic call sign, for confidentiality), at Lancaster Royal Infirmary. Further tests that now I understand to be Weber and Rinne tests, were conducted by "Bravo" one of which involved a vibrating tuning fork being placed on my skull and, as I didn't flinch, I could see by his expression that something was amiss. He then asked me to return the next day for an MRI, which was undertaken on the Thursday of that week. On the Friday he telephoned me at home (you have a gut feeling that it was for not so good news) and he had arranged to see me urgently on Monday morning, 12th March 2007.

After a worrying weekend Carol and I turned up together and "Bravo" issued the words **"Do you want the good news first or the bad news?"** I thought let's get the bad news first. So he said, "The bad news is that you have a brain tumour and the good news is that I believe it to be benign and if so I know a man who can fix it." He then showed me the MRI scan and you could clearly see a large "mass" pressing into and deforming the brainstem (likely to have been the cause for my earlier heart scare). And then I was shown the radiologist's report which said, "The location, morphology and signal characteristics of this lesion indicate a probable diagnosis of an epidermoid tumour."

Why Me? (My Glass Suddenly Emptied).

We were dumbstruck. "Bravo" was such a lovely man and he indicated that he had copied the MRI scan and radiologist report for me to take to Professor "Romeo" in Manchester (the man who could fix it) and he would immediately get his secretary to type up a referral letter. As he lived in Garstang he would hand deliver it to our house. What an absolute hero (his children actually attended the same primary school as ours).

Carol and I then returned to our car and just sat and

cried for an hour to take it all in and to try and decide our next steps, the very first one being to talk to our boys.

So that Monday evening the open letter "popped" through our door as promised. The first line of this letter read: *Dear R, I would be grateful if you could arrange to see this pleasant pharmacist in your rooms for further management.*

The very next morning we telephoned "Romeo's" secretary and explained our situation and read out said letter. She then asked if we could get to Manchester for 12.30 that day as he would see us during his lunch break!

With no more time to waste we set off for Manchester (what a whirlwind).

"Romeo" then confirmed his analysis that I did have an epidermoid tumour and that because of its location at the base of the skull where all the cranial nerves pass through, the "mass effect" had first "knocked out" the most vulnerable nerves i.e. the hearing and balance nerves. He then said it was time to take urgent action as the next nerves which could be affected were the facial nerve (causing facial paralysis) closely followed by the nerves controlling swallowing (which could result in choking to death) and then the chest muscles and heart and lungs. He then explained the nature of the epidermoid and said that it would take two surgeons to undertake such a delicate surgical operation (himself, an ENT surgeon, and a neurosurgeon).

Much to our surprise and consternation he then picked up the phone and casually rang his neurosurgeon colleague ("Sierra") and uttered the words (directed at him), "Hi are you free next Friday? I have a theatre slot available and a gentleman here who needs his epidermoid removing as soon as we can." Carol and I just sat and looked at each other, jaws open in shock and awe.

It was explained that the operation would be at Salford

Royal Hospital NHS, because of the emergency back up available should there be any complications but with costs born (on this occasion by my private insurance). Unfortunately "Sierra" was about to go on holiday and so a date of 29th April 2007 was set. What is an epidermoid tumour? Romeo had told me not to go searching the internet, but of course you do especially if you have a scientific background.

Epidermoids are an unusual form of brain tumour as they are cyst like and usually form in the very early stages of the development of an embryo (usually between third and fifth week of foetal development). They develop when cells that are meant to be skin, hair and nails (epithelial cells) are trapped among the cells that form the brain. An epidermoid has a thin sticky layer (which is alive) of epithelial cells surrounding fluid, keratin and cholesterol. Although usually benign and very slow growing they may grow around and encase cranial nerves and arteries and they strongly adhere to the brain stem. They are most often diagnosed in middle-aged adults (49 years in my case), account for about 0.1% of all brain tumours and about 40% of all epidermoids occur in the cerrobellopontine angle (the location of mine). The CPA is a cistern in the skull base that as well as containing cranial nerves contains cerebrospinal fluid (CSF).

All I then wanted was for this "ticking time bomb" to be removed as soon as possible, yet we had to follow up on a few issues beforehand. Firstly, as we had not already done so, I had to make a will in order to protect Carol and the boys, in the event that I did not make it through such major surgery. We both went to the solicitors and made our wills, we then had to inform our family, friends and employers. A very sobering process. As with all surgical operations (and this was "numero uno" of the 50+ stated at the start of this tale) I had to go for pre-operation checks.

It was at this check that I was told my blood pressure was high (hardly surprising with such stress) and that I needed to reduce it, and as nothing was going to stop me getting "this thing" out of my head I made a GP appointment. My GP's words that still resonate today were, "Any gasman worth his or her salt will be able to work with this and the operation should still go ahead." Further BP checks were done, as well as home monitoring, and it was decided that my BP was acceptable and that I probably suffered from "white coat syndrome" and the operation could proceed as planned.

I went into hospital the night before the Sunday morning operation and we were both seen by the anaesthetist and "Romeo" and "Sierra" to discuss how the operation was to take place the following morning.

A Retro-sigmoid craniotomy (opening in the head behind the ear), was to be performed allowing safe access to the epidermoid for it to be removed safely, however the nature of an epidermoid is that the contents are contained within a very fine capsule and it is not always possible to completely remove the whole of the capsule as it will be adherent to the brain and attempts to do so may cause harm.

I then signed the obligatory consent form and under the section "serious or frequently occurring risks" was written: *Death, stroke, facial numbness and weakness, swallowing difficulties, hydrocephalus, CSF leak, infection and recurrence of cyst.*

I thought "Death" is not just serious it is fatal!

The last three or four of the complications were to plague me for many a year to follow.

On the Sunday morning Carol returned to see me before I went down to theatre and saw "Sierra" again who took her mobile telephone number and said he would call as soon as the operation was complete. Meanwhile I was taken down to theatre, and probably because it was a Sunday, before being taken into the anaesthetics room I was wheeled into another ante-room. I was lying flat on my back in this room and I could see books and files stacked on top of the shelves. One of the files, which I could easily make out, had the title "Procedures to be followed in the event of a death during surgery". Bloody hell, the last thing you wanted to see just before embarking on life-saving major brain surgery! I was really anxious by the time I entered the anaesthetic room and then given the small talk banter, cannulas into the wrist and then off into the land of nod I went.

After many hours of the operation, I was placed in the High Dependency Unit. Poor Carol had been pacing the hospital grounds for all those hours, with help and support from close family and friends (the stress on her I couldn't imagine) when she received a call from "Sierra" stating that the operation had gone well and that they had managed to get at least 99% of the tumour away and that I was in the recovery room and she could see me shortly. As I came around from the anaesthetic I vaguely remember Carol being there holding my hand, and a visit from both surgeons "Romeo" and "Sierra" and we were together, ecstatic with the good news. I recovered in hospital, Carol travelling to Manchester from Garstang every day (which was to become a regular feature over many days, weeks, months and years periodically in the future) and after four days was allowed home (which was also great news as I expected to be in hospital for at least a week).

Chapter 14

Plumbing and Leaks

It was great to return home, but unfortunately after three or so days at home, complications set in. One morning I woke to find my pillow soaked with a clear but halo-tinted stain and a massive severe headache. So an ambulance was called and I was transferred back to Salford Royal Hospital (SRH) where I was diagnosed with meningitis and a cerebrospinal fluid leak (CSF), by which time the pain in my head was unbearable, (it felt like it was going to explode). The CSF was building up and up in my skull and had nowhere to drain.

You can understand why hospitals have restricted opening windows as the pain was so intense I could have easily jumped out of the window to ease it. I would also have gladly used a hammer and nail on my head to relieve the pressure (a feeling I was unfortunately to experience many times to come).

The solution was to have a lumbar puncture and a lumbar drain inserted into the spine to release the pressure (and measure the amount of CSF draining and the actual physical pressure being exerted by its build up inside the skull) and treat the meningitis with antibiotics.

CSF is a watery liquid that continually circulates through the brain's ventricles (hollow cavities) and around the surface of the brain and spinal cord (providing essential nourishment, waste removal and protection to the brain). There is about 150ml of CSF at any one time, and about 500ml is generated every day (and completely renewed about four times over 24 hours). Normally the CSF flows though the ventricles and then finally into the fourth ventricle progressing gently down the spinal cord to eventually be reabsorbed.

A brilliant homeostatic (natural) plumbing and drainage system designed by nature which is hard to replicate artificially and in my case had been disrupted by the brain surgery.

I was in hospital, and after two weeks allowed home again as the head pain had eased and the meningitis resolved, but less than 24 hours later I was back as an emergency case. I had developed severe chest and side pains and couldn't breathe, and that evening a house doctor examined me and asked whether I had been doing any exercise that could have torn a muscle! My reply was acerbic. "You must be joking. I've just been released from your hospital after spending ten days flat on my back." He prescribed painkillers and that was it. Early next morning "Sierra" visited me (as he had been informed that I was back in) and examined me and then said to the staff, "Get this patient straight for a CT scan and X-ray now." He had suspected (which was confirmed by the tests) immediately that I had a pulmonary embolism (clot on the lung). Anticoagulation treatment was initiated, and once again "Sierra" had saved my life, literally. I could have died through the night!

However once again I developed headaches as my CSF began to build up (hydrocephalus). "Sierra" then informed me that I had a non-communicating brain, to which I quipped, "Nothing I haven't been told before, doc", but which actually meant that CSF wasn't flowing between the ventricles and was told that the only solution was to insert a ventriculoperitoneal (VP) shunt (i.e. some artificial plumbing) and hence more surgery.

A VP shunt consists of a catheter (small plastic tube) inserted into the brain ventricles and connected to a valve in the side of the head which is then connected to another catheter which extends into the peritoneal cavity of the abdomen into which the CSF flows to be absorbed.

"Romeo" and "Sierra" also established that my CSF was leaking through my mastoid (an area of bony air cells, located just behind the ear). Thus a mastoidectomy (a procedure performed to remove the mastoid air cells in the skull) was performed. Which again left me feeling rather unwell with an infection gaining hold.

Unfortunately VP shunts can be very problematic and can block, over or under drain and cause bowel perforation (more) of which later. So since my first operation and December 2007 I had a further 12+ operations as "Sierra" tried his utmost to get the correct plumbing system established. "Sierra" also enlisted the help of another neurosurgeon, "Tango" (who specialised in shunts and hydrocephalus). This is an area of medicine that is as complex as it gets.

I was going to theatre so frequently that an operating theatre technician whilst I was in the anaesthetic room joked, "John, we'll have to invite you to the staff Christmas party", which turned out to be a premonition.

Rather than a VP shunt, due to its ongoing problems it was decided to try a more natural approach with an endoscopic third ventriculostomy (ETV). For this once again I had to sign the consent form and once again *Death* was listed as the first serious side effect. "Tango" explained that as part of the operation the endoscopic drilling passed so close to the major brain artery that the blood pressure had to be dropped very low in order to flatten the artery allowing the endoscope to safely pass over it. He explained that if the artery was nicked then it would cause catastrophic bleed and instant death. Very sobering indeed.

As part of the preparation lots of brain CT scans were taken to create a 3D image of the area, and with GPS-like guidance the endoscope created (drilled) a small opening in the bottom of the third ventricle so that CSF can drain further below into the basal cisterns (bypassing the fourth ventricle), and from there into the spinal cord and thus relieve CSF pressure. Unfortunately, this failed and the opening subsequently closed, caused by nasty bacteria entering, resulting in bacterial meningitis, and I became seriously unwell. The experts were trying their best but the enemy was even more resourceful.

The treatment was by the antibiotic "Vancomycin" being directly administered around the brain, via a catheter into the skull. The Vancomycin had to be stored in the fridge and then brought out for a period of time to reach room temperature before administration. However, on some occasions it was administered too cold and what a strange sensation that was as I felt cold liquid going across my brain!

So I found myself in hospital over Christmas, but "Tango" took pity on me and allowed me to go home just for my Christmas dinner with my family, and so Carol drove all the way to Salford to collect me on Christmas morning and then back to Salford after Christmas dinner. It was a fantastic feeling though, to be out and free, albeit too short, and to have an intimate family dinner.

A tricky part of the whole process of getting the "plumbing" correct is knowing whether the massive headaches and fatigue are caused by high Intracranial Pressure (ICP) i.e. too much CSF in brain or low ICP (too little) as the symptoms are so similar. Too low an ICP (depleted CSF) can also be dangerous as in extreme cases it can result in brain collapse.

So when presented with the symptoms a CT scan is undertaken (to establish the state of the ventricles) and possibly also to insert an ICP probe (to physically measure the actual pressure). Under general anaesthetic a very small bore (burr) hole is drilled into the skull and an electronic probe placed inside. This is attached to a lead, and held in place via a bolt in the skull, the lead is then attached to a monitor which itself is attached to an upright moveable stand (nicknamed by me as a "Trolley Dolly"). Over about 48 hours the pressure is recorded day and night, asleep, awake and on the move.

I have had many such operations, many such monitors and spent many hours wandering the hospital and grounds pushing the "Trolley Dolly" on my own or accompanied by Carol, friends and family. In the future such a monitor was to cause an extreme complication and medical emergency for me (more of that later). I didn't realise it in these early days but this was becoming a fixture in my life.

A consequence of being so much on a neuro ward is that you see people much worse off than you and you also experience some strange comings and goings. I remember the nurses saying that patients (when they have a brain disorder) exhibit strange behaviours that are not part of their normal selves.

We had people shouting, being physically violent and trying to escape the ward (for which they had individual 24 hour security, to help the nursing staff). One gentleman drank all the alcohol-based hand sterilisers, so they had to be removed, another kept trying to get into other people's beds (presumably disorientated after loo trips) and we had another who tried to wee on everyone's bed. You had to be forever vigilant which did not bode well for sleeping. You also have to admire the dedication and care of the nursing team, although the very odd one of them could be scary too.

As stated the VP shunting process is artificial plumbing and requires finding the right valves to release the CSF when under pressure but also not to release too much and over drain. Another complication is syphoning, in which the negative pressure at the abdominal (distal) end of the tubing causes a vacuum and starts sucking (syphoning) out more CSF, and so anti-syphon valves are also fitted.

I had many operations trying to find the correct combination and "Tango" stated that he would eventually find the correct combination and regularly consulted with his counterparts at a Liverpool hospital.

Mistakes can happen though, and following one such operation an anti-syphon device had unknowingly been placed upside down. This only came to light when having been sent home, I again suddenly was struck by a massive unbearable headache and taken to Preston Royal Infirmary.

After scans it was then decided (at around 2am) that I should go to theatre for emergency surgery. It was then that the consultant, (who had been "Tango's" registrar who knew me as he had treated me during my previous third ventriculostomy operation) discovered the error and had the device replaced, but unfortunately with a substitute as they did not stock the same device (they are patient specific and normally ordered prior to surgery). Each device has an arrow on the side (as well as part number and serial number, as a register is kept of all implants into a human body). The arrow indicates the direction of flow required (in my case downwards) but the registrar mistook it for "this way up"!

I had to return later to Salford for a replacement valve and "Tango" apologised for the incident and took personal responsibility for it (even though it was the fault of one of his registrars) and asked if I wanted my care to be transferred to Liverpool, but of course I didn't as both "Tango" and "Sierra" had provided such excellent and amazing care.

"Tango" was true to his word and eventually a combination which worked was found, namely a "Codman OSV II" valve (a flow regulation valve operating a three stage, variable resistance mechanism that regulates flow through it) in my head and a "Miethke Shunt Assistant" (a gravitational valve which automatically adjusts its opening pressure to the body position, thus counteracting over drainage in the upright body position) anti-syphon device in my neck. Unbelievable science and medical device ingenuity and many operations.

So for a time I could try and go about and lead an ordinary life outside of hospital. This was not strictly the case as in 2008/9 I underwent surgical procedures (at Blackpool) for inguinal and umbilical hernias (referencing again my training years).

Meanwhile we had acquired a motorhome (which Carol drove as I was not driving) and were able to embark on a few adventures at home and abroad (namely, France, Ireland and even a road trip along the Rhine in Germany). We had to plan our stays where we were not too far from a hospital with neurosurgery facilities (just in case) and we even took with us written "Google" foreign translations of my brief medical history and valve set up.

I also had had a lot of sick absence from work, and because I had not been with the Co-Op for a significant enough period, I soon ran out of sick pay but I was still employed in the hope that I would make a full recovery. My glass was half full again and I was determined for this to be the case.

Chapter 15

Do You Know Who I Am?

I was in regular liaison with the Co-Op HR department, as well as with their Pharmacy Superintendent, and so a very gradual (due to fatigue) return to work was agreed. I was to work in their store in Garstang, under the direct supervision of the pharmacist store manager. I was working in the dispensary labelling medicines and doing computer work. I felt that I did not want to be totally responsible for the "final check" of any prescription dispensed by any member of staff in case a mistake was made which was then not noticed by me. My first thought, as always, was first and foremost patient safety.

Pharmacies had to be under the supervision of the "Pharmacist in Charge" and that person had to be named and logged on a daily basis, for legal responsibility purposes, even if there were three or four pharmacists working only one could be "The Pharmacist in Charge" and I didn't want it to be me, until fully recovered. The Pharmacy Superintendent then believed that even if another registered pharmacist was on the premises then they would be equally responsible for any mistakes made. I did not agree with this and so contacted the General Pharmaceutical Council (GPC) for advice. What a big mistake that turned out to be.

The RPSGB used to be both the statutory legal self-governing and regulatory body as well as the professional advice and training body but, following the Shipman Enquiry, it could not self-regulate and so it divided into the RPSGB (training and advice) and GPC (regulatory) and pharmacists, in order to work, had to be registered (and with their fees paid) with the GPC.

So I telephoned the GPC for advice only and was confronted by sheer un-empathetic officialdom. There was no concern for my health, no suggestions on how to go forward or, indeed, how I could be helped. Nor was there any offer of convalescence (which I'm sure the old original RPSGB would have done). Instead I was told that I would have to be referred to the "Statutory Fitness to Practise Committee".

I then received an official legally written letter informing me that an investigation would take place and that I had to undertake a medical assessment. I only wanted help and here I was being treated like I had committed a crime or malpractice (insensitive to say the least and upsetting after such a career advocating pharmacy).

Anyway the date for my assessment (at Ashton-Under-Lyne) arrived, which I thought would at least be undertaken by a neurological consultant, and so off Carol and I went.

In an office a dour-faced man was sat at a desk facing two empty chairs, upon which Carol and I sat. He didn't even say hello or ask who Carol was and his first words were, "Do you know who I am?" To which I replied, "My assessor on behalf of the GPC."

He then said, "I am Mr X, a forensic clinical psychologist, who has worked on many high profile cases for the Crown, the Home Office and the GPC and it will be my decision as to whether you remain a pharmacist." What utterly ill-mannered pomposity (or words to that effect) I thought. I was both dumbfounded and angry (in equal measure) to be spoken to in this way and that Carol had been ignored.

He then gave me a name and address to remember and said that he would ask me to recite it after asking me a series of questions of which the following is a selection:

Him – "Do you know where you are?"

Me – "OL6 9RL." The post code I had used in the satnav.

Him – "Who is the Prime Minister in charge of the country?"

Me – "Nick Clegg"

Him – "No it isn't"

Me – "Yes it is, it's a coalition government and David Cameron is on holiday and Nick Clegg has assumed charge at the moment."

He then took his watch off and asked:

Him – "Name as many animals as you can in one minute."

Me – I then listed animals in A–Z order starting with aardvark and going through to zebra (via L for lion) and then back up from Z (zebra fish) to A (antelope) but I mentioned lion again.

Him – "You've already said lion."

Me – "Lioness then."

All the time he had to write down my responses.

He then showed me some simple pictures and asked me to name what they were, i.e. boat, anchor, fish etc.

He then threw the paper on the floor and said "pick that up" presumably to check my dexterity so I picked it up thinking to myself *I'll show him dexterity and shove this right where the sun don't shine* but obviously I was more professional about it.

Him – "Are you married?"

Me – "Yes, happily to Carol for 30 years, who is sat here beside me."

Him – "Name as many words as you can beginning with the letter P."

Me – "Perambulate, psychometric, physiological, pathological, pharmacodynamics, paranormal, pharmaceutical, psychological, photosynthesis, paraesthesia, parallelogram, etc. etc." In other words all the longest "p" words I could think of as he had to write them all down.

Him – "What was the name and address I gave you?"

I recited it word for word.

He then had to write his report and so off home we went. In the car Carol complained at how horrible he had been and that she couldn't remember the name and address and that she was thinking of pot, pan, pen etc. for the words.

We then received his report which repeated everything I had told him such as my medical history and the fact that by mid-afternoon I would become fatigued. He then reported my score in his test (I should have it framed really as it will probably never be repeated) which stated, "Scored 100%, which indicates superior cognitive intellect."

The Co-Op had financed legal support for me with my subsequent letters and dealings with the GPC and after many months I received their verdict or as they legally wrote, "Undertakings of Notice of Decision".

Which stated that I could work as a pharmacist but every six months a workplace supervisor was to send a report on my progress and development to the council for an indefinite period, and my consultant needed to send, every six months, a medical report of my condition. The costs for both the supervision and medical reports had to be borne by me (not the council). How draconian and supportive was that?

I had to sign to agree to this if I wished to remain a pharmacist. This was clearly not acceptable to me and so with regret I resigned from the GPC, strictly speaking not true as I had to apply, in writing, to be removed from the Register!

I received a formal letter informing me that "your application has been granted and that you were formally removed from the Register on 14th June 2011".

In essence the end of my role as a humble "sorcerer's apprentice" and 31 years as a registered pharmacist, so sad.

I could no longer call myself a pharmacist (I can use retired pharmacist) and I could no longer use the initials MRPharmS (Member of the Royal Pharmaceutical Society).

Not as bad as Prince Harry not being able to use HRH (but it certainly felt like it to me). **Why me?**

Chapter 16

Why Carol? (My Heavenly Angel of Darlington)

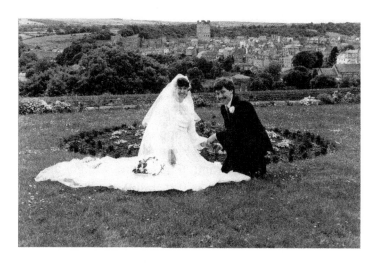

So I became a full-time domestic engineer (at home). My new job competencies included all washing, cooking, cleaning and ironing as Carol was working full time.

In late 2012 Carol began to have walking difficulties at work and unfortunately she experienced several falls, so it was off to the GP and a referral to an orthopaedic consultant as hip arthritis was suspected, and later confirmed. We just thought this was normal wear and tear, however she also started to drop things and developed difficulty with writing and holding a pen. Carpal Tunnel Syndrome (in which pressure on a nerve in the wrist causes pain and numbness in the hand and fingers) was suspected and Carol was referred for electric nerve tests on the wrist and arm.

This involved a technician sticking fine needles (with electrodes attached) into various positions along the arm and the resulting electrode potential measured. The technician then declared that it wasn't CTS and that there was a higher function disorder involved. This immediately triggered alarm bells in my brain resulting in extreme concern and many thoughts and reasons (which I kept to myself, initially). I was thinking please don't let it happen to Carol, please don't let it be a brain tumour, please don't let it be neuro muscular dystrophy. My mind was in overdrive.

So, Carol was then referred to a neurologist at Preston Royal Infirmary, who looked at her medical history and conducted a physical examination and said that he wanted to arrange a brain MRI scan and take a CSF sample via a lumbar puncture there and then. Here we go again, I thought, but this time it was Carol, not me (and that hurt me much worse emotionally).

He indicated that the sample taken had to be analysed and he would "get back to us". We then had an agonising wait for weeks until eventually Carol telephoned the hospital and she was told that the CSF sample had been lost (such incompetence) and she would have to return for another lumbar puncture to be done and a new sample taken. In the meanwhile the MRI had been undertaken.

We returned, to see the consultant on 3rd Feb 2013 to be given the bad news that Carol had developed Primary Progressive Multiple Sclerosis. There were more tears as we knew that this was a disease that was only going to worsen. I was gutted and I took the news badly. Anybody would. We were both devastated. I could pragmatically handle my own diagnosis but was lost as how to cope with Carol's and could only hope that the speed of deterioration would be very slow so that we could try and lead as much of a normal life as possible.

MS is an autoimmune condition and occurs when something goes wrong with the immune system and it mistakenly attacks a healthy part of the body – in this case, the brain. The immune system attacks the myelin sheath (a protective layer around the nerves) and damages and scars the sheath, and potentially the underlying nerves, meaning that messages travelling along the nerves become slow or disrupted.

I felt that what had happened to me and, indeed, us both had caused extreme stress which had contributed (I felt guilty). The consultant advised (when I asked) that stress can exacerbate symptoms but not cause MS and exactly what causes MS is unknown. Most experts think a combination of genetic and environmental factors is involved. Currently there is no cure for MS but a number of treatments can help control symptoms, yet this is currently limited for PPMS. Hopefully, before there is too much deterioration, we live in hope that a cure or delaying mechanism can be found by science, particularly in the field of gene therapy and treatments. I just kept thinking, "**Why Carol?**"

All her life (since I have known her), Carol has dedicated herself to helping and supporting others i.e. as a youth leader, beavers leader, cub-scouts leader, special needs learning support assistant, development officer for offenders, as a learning and support senior lecturer for adults with both physical and mental development needs and finally as my carer.

Glass empty again, it is just not fair and yet there are people worse off than us as we have each other and a great network support of friends and family who have been "there" for us.

In March 2017 we decided to move once again, this time only to the opposite end of Garstang. We downsized into a bungalow in order to prepare (whilst we were still physically able to do so) for whatever the future may befall us, particularly in respect to Carol's mobility.

In June 2018, at the age of 60, Carol's MS (mainly due to extreme fatigue) resulted in her early retirement from work.

Unfortunately more was to happen, for us both, which would further add to the stress.

Carol's dad, (Tony) was diagnosed with Vascular Dementia (circa 2014) which, after several falls (resulting in hospitalisations and several care home residencies), contributed to his passing (7th March 2019, aged 83).

He was such a gentle, fun-loving father who supported and loved his family (and dogs) above all else. Traits which Carol has clearly inherited.

Her mam (Margaret) was subsequently diagnosed with Alzheimer's disease (circa 2016) and with strong will and determination managed (until very recently), with daily carers, to remain in the matrimonial home until late summer 2022.

She then required 24 hour nursing home care. Unfortunately, at the time of writing this page, she passed away peacefully yesterday (29th October 2022, aged 88).

Margaret was the matriarch of the family, fun loving and absolutely dedicated to her immediate family and friends. My mother-in-law and I enjoyed great "banter" over the 48 years that I knew her, in particular my reference to her as WWN (Wicked Witch of the North) which she shared with such good humour. Over the years I have bought her many a witch and related memorabilia, also she would knit witches for me and even sign birthday and Christmas cards with witch logos.

Margaret, like Tony, will be greatly missed, much loved and remembered by us all.

It is my belief that she has cast a loving and caring

spell over us all, that will never be broken.

Dementia (an umbrella term really, of dementia types which includes Alzheimer's 60–80%, Vascular 5–10%, Lewy Body 5–10%, Frontotemporal 5–10%, Other 5–10% incl. Huntington's and Parkinson's, and mixed) leads to a decline in memory, reasoning or other thinking skills. It has such a massive impact on individuals, their families, social care and healthcare provision and the decline is so cruel to witness.

MS is a degenerative condition, progression of which is usually measured by EDSS (Expanded Disability Status Scale), a functional system (FS) represented by a network of neurons in the brain with responsibility for particular tasks. Each FS is scored on a scale of 0 (no disability) to 5 or 6 (more severe disability). EDSS steps 5.0 to 9.5 are defined by the impairment to walking.

Carol's has now, unfortunately, progressed to 6.0, which represents a requirement of a walking aid (cane, crutch etc.) in order to walk about 100m with or without resting.

We personally assess her progression by how far into town she is able to walk without stopping; this is getting shorter and shorter and it is frustrating for Carol and deeply upsetting for me to witness (we used to love walking the fells, hills and dales together). Sometimes the spasms are so severe that all movement stops and she freezes and has to wait for muscular action to return.

In the words of our boys' primary school motto we are **"Stronger Together"** and as such whatever "comes our way" we will face and deal with together. Carol is my heavenly Angel of Darlington.

The words of the song "Music" by John Miles sums it up for me if you substitute all the words "music" with the name Carol.

Chapter 17

Bust a Gut

2013 was to be our Annus horribilis (latin – meaning "horrible year") to pinch a quote from our late Queen (Elizabeth II).

This year I spent most of a glorious summer in Preston Royal Infirmary, again very ill.

In late May I was admitted twice due to severe abdominal pain, which was initially thought to be the result of a hernia. So I was discharged, only to return again with abdominal pain and they undertook abdominal keyhole surgery (still thinking it was an umbilical hernia, which had shown up on a ultrasound scan). However, no hernia was found but a lot of adhesive tissue (from previous surgeries) was found and removed and I was discharged again.

But in June I was admitted again (in agony) and an ultrasound was conducted upon which the consultant radiographer was concerned and so sent me for an abdominal MRI which showed a concerning mass in the right hand side of my abdomen. At around 3am the pain was so severe that they took me straight into emergency theatre.

Initially the mass was to be removed via keyhole surgery but this proved to be too dangerous and so a mid-line laparotomy (a long surgical abdominal incision stretching from the belly button to pubic area) was performed. The mass (which was dead tissue i.e. necrotic omentum) was removed together with my appendix. The omentum (a large adipose tissue layer which stores fat and plays key roles in immune regulation and tissue

166

regeneration) had been caught up in the furthermost (distal) end of my shunt.

The shunt was not removed but re-sited from the right side of my abdomen to the left side. Post-operative pain was extreme and I was put on strong analgesia, firstly morphine (which caused vomiting and hallucinations), then fentanyl (a much stronger synthetic opioid) via a syringe driver. I then developed a further complication from which ensued a prolonged stay.

My abdomen was getting bigger and bigger like a massive space hopper and a nasal gastric tube had to be inserted and kept in place for weeks (not a pleasant procedure at all) to release litres and litres of green bile built up inside the stomach. I had developed paralytic ileus (a major obstruction from the stomach into the intestines) with which no food or liquids could pass from the stomach to the intestines. I could not eat or drink anything so a PICC line (peripherally inserted central catheter) was inserted. This is a small feeding tube which is passed through a vein in the arm and passing directly into the heart along which total parental nutrition (TPN) is sent. TPN contains a mixture of protein, carbohydrates, glucose, fat, vitamins and minerals and is made up on a patient by patient basis depending upon an individual's requirements assessed by blood test. The bag is usually hung from a moveable stand and covered with a red bag to protect from certain wavelengths of light. So again I could be seen pushing around a "Trolley Dolly" but this time with a red handbag.

I was in for weeks and Carol visited me every day, bless her, as did family and friends.

Now I needed to get things moving, literally. I had researched an article that chewing gum might ease the paralysis (in theory fooling the intestines into thinking food was on its way) and so I began chewing gum all the time. Well it must have worked because the blockage stopped and I regained bowel function as well as the ability to eat and drink and so was discharged. I had regularly, during this inpatient stay, asked for intervention by the neuro team but alas to no avail and it was all dealt with by the gastro team.

Shortly after discharge I was re-admitted (Preston again) with renewed abdominal pain this time in my left side (surprise, surprise as the shunt tubing had been moved). An abdominal X-ray revealed further coiling of the distal tubing, and the neurosurgery team were involved this time.

If you are thinking that patient's opinions should be listened to more respectfully by the experts, so do I. There is no doubt I am here today because of their dedication, determination and expertise, but… nobody is so perfect they know everything.

I was taken to theatre this time under a local anaesthetic, by neurosurgeon "Golf". This was certainly a traumatic experience as I saw a laser knife (which reminded me of a scene in the James Bond film, *Goldfinger*) make an incision in my abdomen and "Golf" then tried to pull the shunt tubing out of the abdominal cavity at which I screamed and screamed in pain and the theatre nurse asked "Golf" to stop as the shunt was firmly coiled and anchored and going nowhere so the shunt was tied off inside the abdomen.

I then went down to theatre again the next day (under general anaesthetic) for the VP shunt to be converted to a ventriculopleural shunt (the distal end of the tubing placed inside the pleural space of the lung). However, I then developed extreme severe right-sided chest pain (I couldn't breathe or move) due to irritation of the diaphragm so back in theatre again the shunt was externalised to drain inside a container outside the body.

I then became infected with a gramme negative bacterium resulting in bacterial meningitis again and subsequent intravenous antibiotic treatment. Once this had cleared a trial was carried out to clamp the shunt (to see if the non-drainage then caused high ICP) and to test whether I still required a shunt. (I was always confirmed as being shunt dependant at Salford.)

It appeared that I did not go into high pressure or exhibit headaches (the exact reason will become apparent further in the story as investigated subsequently by Salford) and tolerated the clamping and so the shunt was tied off and placed inside the body in the upper neck (supraclavicular) region and then I was discharged home.

This episode does not end here as at the end of 2013 I developed an abscess at the tied-off end in the neck. This required a further local procedure to drain the abscess and remove some further shunt tubing. The catheter tubing in my brain, OSV II valve and shunt assistant device were left in place (in case later required) together with a short end of the peritoneal catheter left in the mid-neck. What a year! And I survived it, yet caused Carol more stress. Was 2014 going to be any better?

Chapter 18

Dripping Tap and Blown Gaskets

In the spring of 2014 I became aware of an abnormal taste and a sensation of fluid running down the back of my throat as well as intermittently coming out of my nose. This manifested itself when "pottering around" and leaning forward, when I would almost always have a watery discharge (dripping tap) out of my nostrils.

I was again admitted to Preston in June 2014 with severe headache photophobia and neck stiffness, and my CSF showed a high white cell count. I was thus treated (yet again, unbelievable I know) for bacterial meningitis with two weeks of IV antibiotics but with no further neurosurgical involvement at this time!

I was released from Preston hospital but my nasal discharge continued, and I was continually aware of fluid either at the back of my throat or coming out of my nose, together with a feeling of a "fuzzy head" and disorientation (low ICP symptoms). I then contacted Salford Royal Hospital, via "Sierra's" medical secretary.

Then "Sierra" telephoned me personally, at home (a true indication of his brilliant care, expertise and bedside manner). He told me that he had discussed my case with the neurosurgical multi-disciplinary team and that he had reached a hypothesis as to the reasons for the events.

He believed that I am always shunt dependant and that my apparent tolerance to the tying off of my VP shunt was in fact misleading due to the development of a spontaneous skull-based fistula (hole) which acted to decompress any rise in intracranial pressure (in my words, a blown gasket) and the development of bacterial meningitis was related to the fistula (that is, if fluid can leak out of the skull then bacteria can get in).

I told him that I was just about to go on holiday in our motorhome, that very day, to Dorset and he indicated that, as it was in the UK and there were good neurosurgery hospitals nearby, we could go on holiday and if any complications arose I should go straight to the hospital and ask their neurosurgical team to contact him urgently.

In the meanwhile he would arrange for further tests at Salford on my return. Fortunately there weren't any complications whilst on holiday and we had a leisurely and quiet time trying to relax.

Immediately on return from holiday I went to Salford for scans and a cisternogram (more plumbing terminology).

A cisternogram (nuclear medicine imaging) involves injection of a radioactive material into the CSF in the spine via a lumbar puncture and using real-time X-ray (fluoroscopy) to ensure accuracy. This also meant lying very still for an hour whilst the radioactive substance moved through my CSF.

*

Then the fun began, to actively view the leak in real-time various imaging of the spine and brain is undertaken. This involved lying face down with the trolley bed tipped down at an angle of at least 45 degrees, with my head almost on the floor and my feet in the air whilst being wheeled around the hospital to different CT scan and MRI machines. In total over a four hour period I had two CT scans and two MRI scans. Along with the dozens and dozens of scans in total over time it is a wonder that I don't light up in the dark.

The results indicated that a leak was suspected in the cribriform plate (a portion of bone located at the base of the skull). "Sierra" and "Tango" and another endoscopic skull-based surgeon "Kilo" discussed the best course of action, which was to have two further neurosurgical operations. You can't walk around with a leak in your head after all.

The first priority surgery was to place a renewed VP shunt to provide CSF diversion and the second, separate operation to repair the skull base defect (plug the hole). The hole couldn't just be plugged without the shunt in place as it would just blow again!

The second operation was undertaken by "Kilo" and again was very risky as it involved a transnasal repair with the aid of a fat graft and nasal septal flap (tissue reconstruction). In other words an endoscope is inserted right up through the nose to the base of the skull and fat (taken from the thigh) is grafted onto the skull base.

The operation was successful in plugging the leak and again life saving and yet it has left me with a long term deficit in that I have permanently lost my sense of taste and smell (so I have great empathy for those suffering this during long Covid).

This loss was due to the endoscope damaging the olfactory bulb (a structure located in the forebrain that receives neural input about odours detected by cells in the nasal cavity) high up the nose. So now I had lost my hearing and balance nerves in the left hand side and now also my sense of taste and smell, but I'm still alive to enjoy life (glass half full again).

In the immortal words of the '66 world cup "they think it's all over" well sorry it isn't.

Everything was appearing to settle down until 2017 with one planned surgery and one which had drastic consequences.

Chapter 19

BAHA

A consequence of being unable to hear in one ear was that I found it difficult to hear and talk in large groups of people and in noisy situations. Also, when walking along a road (without stereo hearing) I could not differentiate which direction traffic was approaching, and when my only good ear became blocked (as it does with wax regularly) then I couldn't hear anything at all. My balance would also suffer badly.

I was referred to Audiology (Lancaster Royal Infirmary), who trialled cross-over hearing aids which picks up sound in the left aid and transmits it, electronically via blue tooth, to the aid in my right ear. The sounds were then passed down a fine tube into the right ear and picked up by the hearing nerve (the only one remaining). The only problem with this is that the tube in my right ear blocked any sound I could hear normally with that ear.

I was then referred to an ENT consultant who told me that I qualified (due to my medical conditions) under the NHS for a BAHA device. BAHA is not a sound made by a baby or a sheep but is actually a bone anchored hearing aid (made and developed by Cochlear™). This would involve more surgery.

A BAHA is composed of two parts:

1. **External part**: the box, **a sound processor** and external microphone device which receives sounds from the environment converting them into vibrations. The vibrations then get transmitted to the embedded implant.

2. **Internal part**: the **titanium implant**. When

receiving vibrations from the outside mechanism the left sided implant vibrates the surrounding bone (skull), transmitting sound waves through the skull into the inner ear (right side) which then stimulates the hair cells and activates the right-sided auditory nerve.

To surgically implant the BAHA hearing aid, the ENT surgeon installs the titanium implant (about 4mm in length) into the mastoid bone behind the ear and, over time, the titanium integrates with the bone. The sound processor external device is then attached or removed by the patient via a clipping, press-stud-like mechanism (push fitted onto an abutment).

The actual surgery (March 2017) was painless but nonetheless slightly traumatic as it was conducted under local anaesthetic. Whilst you don't feel the pain you do feel the pressure and intense vibrations as your head is drilled and the implant screwed deeply into position. You can also feel the blood and fluids oozing down your head (sorry for the graphic detail but it felt like a Black and Decker drill was being used on my skull).

I am aware that anyone reading this will, by now, be wondering why and how I submit to all these surgeries which must be starting to sound like high-tech medicine's answer to the medieval torture chamber. I can assure you I don't make these decisions lightly. The glass half full analogy is the answer. Fate has delivered me an unusually full set of challenges. I can respond in two ways: I can give up and take an easier root or, I can take advantage of the interventions offered by modern medicine to lead to the most normal life possible. As you can tell, I have been blessed with an exceptional life partner and my sons bring me great happiness. In return, I want to do everything I can to support them. Agreeing to medical help is a logical imperative.

After the operation and a few days recuperation we

then went away in our motorhome to Buxton in Derbyshire for a well-deserved break. Whilst on holiday the area around the implant (abutment) became red, inflamed and infected with pus and I developed a headache. So Carol, her sister (who lived close by) and I visited Buxton Cottage Hospital.

They inspected me and requested my medical history (which took some considerable time to explain) and said that they needed to seek advice from the nearest A&E hospital (which was miles away in Stockport, Greater Manchester). The ENT consultant at the said Stepping Hill Hospital informed them that I needed to come to their A&E department straight away and they would be waiting for me.

Stepping Hill had been all over the national and local TV news for an incident which began in July 2011, three patients were found to have been unlawfully killed by poisoning at the hospital (allegedly via IV infusions). So we drove there with a natural degree of trepidation. But there is at least one bad egg in any barrel and this was no reflection on the brilliant hard work undertaken by the massive majority of staff.

My heart did flutter as we approached the entrance and saw the view that had been plastered over our TV screens and I jokingly said to Carol, "I hope they don't give me an IV drip."

The consultant and staff were absolutely brilliant, kind and empathetic but our hearts did jump when I was told I needed to be admitted for 24 hours to have an IV infusion of antibiotics.

Scans had been completed and they thought that the infection was superficially localised but that I needed the infusion to ensure it didn't develop any further especially with my history. Carol went to her sister's to stay overnight and I was discharged the next day, after being nursed very well.

So the summer progressed agreeably and Carol and I had a lovely holiday in Le Bus (our motor home) on Jersey.

I even made my son Sean's stag weekend which was an event indeed. About 30 of us travelled down by coach, setting off early after breakfast and beer at the "local" to Bournemouth dressed in our obligatory pink coloured stag shirts with slogans written on the back; mine was "Big John". Which was all well and dandy until we discovered, when we arrived, that it was Gay Pride weekend in Bournemouth. In the immortal words "whatever happens on stag stays on the stag".

As we moved into autumn I started to develop headaches, dizziness and light headedness once again and so in early November I was admitted to Salford Royal for ICP monitoring in order to determine shunt malfunction and whether the symptoms were a result of high or low pressure (another date with the "Trolley Dolly").

Chapter 20

Heaven and Hell

"Heaven and Hell" is a Black Sabbath album track written by the late Ronnie James Dio and if you know the lyrics (or are able to look them up) then you may find them to perhaps be poignant for the next event.

Shortly after the probe insertion I became so unwell that my temperature rocketed to about 40 degrees and I became delirious and confined to my ward bed. I can vaguely remember Carol telling the nurse that I was vacant and "not with it". They both thought I was experiencing petit mal: absence seizures involving brief, sudden lapses of consciousness and looking like I was staring into space for a few seconds. I can't remember these at all, but Carol recognised the symptoms through her experience at work.

What was to follow (which I vividly remember) was many grand mal seizures (generalised tonic-clonic seizures) with violent muscle contractions throughout my body, and it felt as if every muscle was in spasm. These were preceded by a vision of a red, horned cloven-footed beast (I truly thought it was the devil) dragging me violently by my arms and shaking me. I remember screaming out "get him off me. He's dragging me away" as the spasms began to hurt. I am not religious and my scientific mind tells me that the very high temperature was causing misfiring in the brain synapses and that this was not real, yet it appeared vividly to me that way.

The seizures got more frequent and violent and on one occasion I felt that I had been dragged into a very dark tunnel. Then a light appeared at the end and an infant child appeared directing me another way. I like to think that if this was real then it was Our Ross saving me. But my scientific mind tells me that it was perhaps an illusion brought about by the drugs that were being pumped into me to control the seizures. Perhaps I had watched too many horror films and my brain was misfiring memories. I am not inventing this, it really happened and felt so real to me and I have only ever spoken about this to Carol, but now you know too and I am opening up, warts and all. Even in these enlightened days we all know men still don't talk, but we are starting to write. Most people have never experienced this kind of psychotic reality, so just pause for a second to imagine what it is like. At the time it feels 100% real. The question "what is real?" is fundamental to both psychology and philosophy. It is what you believe in at the time.

In a gap between these seizures I remember being accompanied by an ICU nurse with an emergency back pack to a scanner and all the time hoping that I didn't have a seizure on the way to or indeed inside the scanner. The seizures were getting worse and I was admitted into the neurological intensive care unit. Carol was really scared, worried and stressed.

I spent three days in ICU though I can only remember snippets as I was really delirious by then, and I thought that I was in a spaceship being attended to by humanoid robots whose every movement was slow and in a delayed time sequence. It seemed that they were monitoring me from a console unit and speaking to me via a microphone.

Their step approach to me also sounded very loud as boots seemed to be dragged across a metal grid.

Carol was later to describe to me that the unit was ultra-modern with individual pods for patients and the console was a large angled desk at the end of the bed with a large paper chart upon which every detail (including blood results) was manually written by my individual ICU specialist nurse, but I was still convinced I had been in a space ship.

Of course they brought the seizures under control with high doses of anti-epileptic medication and I was put on an intensive IV antibiotic regime which would have to be given for six weeks.

The consultant informed me that a Klebsiella Pneumonia infection had caused a deep abscess within the frontal lobe area of the brain which had triggered the seizures. They informed me that as the seizures were controlled, I could go home for Christmas if a district nurse team could be found to daily administer the IV infusions. This proved more difficult than envisaged to organise because we lived between three different Primary Care funding groups and funds were not readily available.

Fortunately a nurse specialist was tenacious in getting this organised. The NHS, like all organisations, depends as much on these individual heroes as it does on its systems. And so, rather than have nurses come to me, it was agreed for the remaining four weeks (including Christmas day and New Year's Day) that Carol would drive me daily to a specialist unit at Preston Royal Hospital for the infusions, so that I could spend Christmas at home.

The team at Preston were excellent and so very caring and, as I was on long term treatment, they arranged for a PICC line to be inserted into a vein in my arm and then into my heart so that the antibiotics could be infused without the need for an IV cannula (which would have needed replacement every three days). My bloods were checked twice weekly and blood pressure daily until I was eventually clear of the infection.

Mid-January 2018 I was released from their care, and

my glass was half full again and we could begin some normality.

It was then back to Salford for a review and a further CT scan of the abscess. I was subsequently told that I had focal epilepsy and that I would have to take anti-epileptic drugs for the rest of my life and also told to inform the DVLA and not to drive. (Glass cracked again.)

Apparently the abscess (which had been excised in another operation) had caused deep-seated scarring which is epileptogenic (meaning it has an enhanced probability to generate recurrent seizures).

I am under annual review for my hydrocephalus at Salford and with Preston (as local) for my epilepsy and I know that I can contact the relevant medical secretaries should any need arise. After three years (2020) with appropriate medical reports and no seizures I was able to have my driving licence returned and am able again to support Carol with driving to help her fatigue. The good news is that "Sierra" believes that there is no evidence of any residual epidermoid and therefore no signs of re-growth.

My last operation in May 2021 (of less serious concern) was a total left hip replacement, necessary as a result of wear and tear (osteoarthritis), probably brought about due to all that sport (squash, cricket, volleyball and windsurfing) which alas is no more.

Since 2007 I have taken up learning to play the guitar (I have quite a collection, even building a couple from scratch) though I am a forever beginner.

Due to my valves, shunt, BAHA and artificial hip I feel like the *Six Billion Dollar Man* (for those of you who can remember the '70s TV series). If you are too young it was about Steve Austin, an astronaut who was seriously injured when his spaceship crashed. He then underwent government-sanctioned surgery, which rebuilt several of

Steve's body parts with machine parts, making him cyborg like, with superhuman strength (the latter of course does not apply to me).

Chapter 21

A Day Lost (TGA)

My scariest moments in time were those experienced during my epileptic seizures and yet another frightening period (the irony is that today, as I write it is All Hallows Eve) was October 8th 2021, a day in which the hours between 9am and 6pm were completely lost to me. I am able to describe this event only because Carol has recalled it to me.

Apparently I drove Carol and our two grandchildren a couple of miles across town, dropped them off at their Zumbini class (a baby and toddler exercise class) and then went home with the intentions of collecting them, once the class had finished. After the class finished Carol (as there was no sign of me or the car) telephoned me at home. I recognised her voice but had no recollection of dropping them off, and I could not even remember where the venue was located. Carol then gave me directions and somehow I drove the car to the venue, then just remained in the car looking vague and bewildered and it was at this point that she told me to change seats and she drove us all home.

During the afternoon I just sat "Zombie like" in my armchair, repetitively asking her whether or not I had taken my medication. I had also asked why we had received post for our son Lewis only to be told he had been living with us for three weeks, whilst waiting to move into his new house. I just couldn't remember or even evaluate this information. At this point Carol became very concerned and contacted our GP, and because of my medical history they told us to go straight to Preston hospital A&E. This was during Covid restrictions and as such you were only allowed admittance on your own following a temperature check. Because I could not recall the day's events, Carol was given permission for entry too.

When we saw the doctors, Carol had to relay the events of the day yet bizarrely I could recount my full medical history to them. A neuro consultant was called who conducted the usual neurological tests and requested blood tests, an X-ray, CT scan and brain EEG to establish if it was an issue with my shunt, an epilepsy seizure or some other cause.

We spent the whole night in the hospital and returned home (at 6am) due to the facts that the shunt was operational and the CT scan and EEG did not highlight anything of concern.

I was advised not to drive until further notice pending further investigations and a MRI brain scan.

The event was later to be diagnosed as Transient Global Amnesia (TGA).

TGA *is an episode of confusion that comes on suddenly in a person who is otherwise alert. This confused state isn't caused by a more common neurological condition, such as epilepsy or stroke.*

During an episode of TGA, a person is unable to create new memory, so the memory of recent events disappears. You can't remember where you are or how you got there. You may not remember anything about what's happening right now. You may keep repeating the same questions because you don't remember the answers you've just been given. You may also draw a blank when asked about things that happened a day, month or even a year ago.

You do remember who you are, you can follow simple directions and you recognise the people you know well.

Episodes of TGA always get better slowly, although not serious it can be frightening.

Other symptoms which help diagnosis are

- *short duration of less than 24 hours*
- *gradual return of memory*
- *no recent head injury*
- *no signs of seizures during the period of amnesia*
- *no history of active epilepsy*

The cause of TGA is unknown but risk factors include

- *Age i.e. 50 years and older*
- *History of migraines*

All in all just another event in my neurological portfolio, although a frightening one.

Epilogue

Having read this story you might well be tempted to ask yourself the question "How has he coped with such trauma and tragedy and could I have done so?" My answer is simple: as humans, we all have the innate ability to deal with trauma and tragedy in our own way (it is how our brains are wired).

I could have answered with some "pyscho-babble" read during my management training and official assessment, described earlier. Was it the fact that my Myers–Briggs personality profile of ESFP (Extroversion, Sensing, Feeling, Perceiving) i.e. the "Entertainer/Performer" (describing me as a spontaneous, energetic, outgoing, friendly, accepting, exuberant lover of life and people, enjoying working with others to make things happen, and an enthusiastic person – life is never boring around them)?

You can make what you will of this description but like a horoscope you always "see" something in it. I also wonder whether it is a result of Nature or Nurture or, both.

Nature – I am wired to be a "fighter" due to genes inherited from my Middlesbrough relatives.

Nurture – Is it a result of my upbringing, development, education and past experiences?

Is it that another such assessment showed me to be a pragmatist and activist, or is it simply that I am a Yorkshireman?

What I do know is that I draw in my energy from the love and support of Carol and my family.

Another coping mechanism has been my joy of music, and during all those lonely hours spent in hospital/s and when my head wasn't "banging" with pain I would listen to a selection of tracks from the 5000 or so stored in my phone.

In the words of the rock band Uriah Heep some are *Very 'Eavy, Very 'Umble* with a variety of genres.

With plenty of spare time I have managed to "whittle down" this 5000 to my top ten favourites. They have been chosen because of their lyrics, melodies and "singing" guitar riffs, and I list them for you, in reverse order (if you so desire, listen to one or two you may be surprised even if it is not normally your style of music):

10 –"Parisienne Walkways" – Gary Moore

9 – "Layla (unplugged version)" – Eric Clapton

8 – "Free Bird" – Lynyrd Skynyrd

7 – "Soldier of Fortune" – Deep Purple

6 – "Bird of Paradise" – Snowy White

5 – "Changes" – Black Sabbath

4 – "Stairway To Heaven" – Led Zeppelin

3 – "Brothers in Arms" – Dire Straits

2 – "Life is Too short" (Acoustic version) – Scorpions

1 – "Unspoken Words" – Status Quo

You may notice that no Beatles, Adele, Tamla Motown or Meatloaf tracks are listed above, but they do appear on my phone.

I wrote the following poem as an entry in a 50 word literature competition about light:

Some marvel at the light of sun or moon beam

Yet, for me it is the light in a hospital, seen or unseen

The focus of the CT scanner discovering the tumour in my brain

The magnified light and laser in the skilled surgeons hand enabling me to live again

It summarises for me my hospital journeys.

My life has not been all trauma and we have experienced many good times including holidays, the weddings (and stag dos) of both our sons, the birth of our grandson and granddaughter (who add a drop to the glass every time we see them), special birthdays, our special wedding anniversaries (silver, and ruby) and many other family celebrations. I could go on and on but I am so glad and blessed to have survived to experience such wonderful occasions. Nobody knows what life will throw at us next (just look at the Covid pandemic) but with love and support and a half full glass we can get through it together. **Stronger Together**.

I started writing this book to share my life story starting from my Middlesbrough roots, all the way through to becoming a patient pharmacist followed by a pharmacist patient. I hope in some small way, with my heart on my sleeve, that I have done so.

This has not been about round the world sailing or an Everest or arctic expedition but it has been challenging nonetheless both physically and mentally as life can be. (Nobody said it was a bed of roses did they?)

Counselling for trauma, tragedy and loss is important and if it does not seek you out then please seek it out. Please talk and share your thoughts and concerns, even in your darkest moments. Remember and celebrate all those close to you, who have passed on.

Take account for your health – **habenda ratio valetudinis**.

Acknowledgements

Life would have not been the same without Carol who for 49 years (so far) has been my best friend, my soul mate, my rock, my confidante and, on many an occasion, my carer. I feel so blessed that she is always by my side and I love her so dearly.

Throughout my continued illness we have both been supported by all of our close families (especially our two sons Lewis and Sean) as well as special friends.

The support has been in many forms both physically (visiting me in hospital, at home, accompanying me to hospital appointments etc.) and mentally (giving much love, time, emotional support and generally "being there" for us both).

So many to name and yet their deeds and actions have been so special to us both and we are so grateful and thank them dearly from the "bottom of our hearts".

I would also like to thank all the various hospital, medical and nursing teams as well as our general practitioners who have given so much care and expertise to us both.

Thanks to the multi-disciplinary neurosurgery team at Salford Royal Hospital including "Sierra", "Romeo", "Tango" and "Kilo" who have, without any doubt, saved my life. Thanks also goes to their medical secretaries, who are unsung heroes too.

Whilst writing about Salford Royal Hospital the words of "Smoke on the Water" by the rock band Deep Purple spring to mind. But,with apologies to Deep Purple, my mind changes the chorus to:

Salford Royal Hospital, a fire in the sky
Salford Royal Hospital

Anecdotally whilst on ward "A3" builders had caused

a small fire, together with resulting smoke, and the ward was evacuated, and yet the key words for me, in respect of all my inpatient stays there were that no matter what I got out of this, I knew I'd never forget.

Thank you all, live life
John Atkinson

About the Author

John Atkinson was born in Middlesbrough, Yorkshire and graduated as a Bachelor of Pharmacy (Hons) from the University of Bradford registering as a Pharmacist with the Royal Pharmaceutical Society of Great Britain.

He worked in many locations throughout the UK as a Pharmacist, Store and Senior Manager for the national Boots the Chemists, United Co-operatives and miscellaneous pharmacy chains and independents.

This included representation on multiple professional bodies such as the Company Chemists Association, Local Pharmaceutical Committees (Morecambe Bay and Durham) and even represented the RPSGB at a Labour Party Conference.

During a 25-year-plus career he was responsible for the training and tutoring of numerous pre-registration Pharmacy graduates, dispensing technicians and assistants.

His hobbies include league volleyball (player, coaching and refereeing), windsurfing, walking and motor-caravanning.

A Patient Pharmacist is his debut book, inspired by a desire to share life experiences – a story of love and support in a war against the odds.

www.blossomspringpublishing.com

Printed in Great Britain
by Amazon

24731380R00111